# 30-day BootCamp: Your Ultimate Weight Loss Plan

# 30-day BootCamp: Your Ultimate Weight Loss Plan

Valerie Orsoni-Vauthey
Celebrity Coach; Founder
MyPrivateCoach.com

iUniverse, Inc.
New York Lincoln Shanghai

30-day BootCamp: Your Ultimate Weight Loss Plan
Copyright © 2006 by Valerie Orsoni-Vauthey

iUniverse books may be ordered through booksellers or by contacting:

iUniverse
2021 Pine Lake Road, Suite 100
Lincoln, NE 68512
www.iuniverse.com
1-800-Authors (1-800-288-4677)

The information contained in this book is provided for general informational purposes only. It is not intended as and should not be relied upon as medical advice. The information may not apply to you and before you use any of the information provided in the site, you should contact a qualified medical, dietary, fitness or other appropriate professional. If you utilize any information provided in this book, you do so at your own risk and you specifically waive any right to make any claim against *30-day BootCamp* as the result of the use of such information.

ISBN-13: 978-0-595-38006-0 (pbk)
ISBN-13: 978-0-595-82377-2 (ebk)
ISBN-10: 0-595-38006-9 (pbk)
ISBN-10: 0-595-82377-7 (ebk)

Printed in the United States of America

# Table of Contents

# What People Are Saying

"Sensible, easy and pragmatic. A must-buy for anybody looking to become fit and thin in a healthy, realistic way: one day at a time."
*Steve Kemp—three-time Decathlon World Champion—Olympic athlete*

"At last, a practical, realistic, easy-to-follow and no-nonsense weight-loss book. If you want to get in shape for your date, this is a sure bet."
*Sandra Harmon—"New York Times" bestselling author of "Elvis and Me", "Getting to I DO" and "Staying Married and Loving It"—#1 Celebrity Love Coach*

"Useful, practical, real-life tips that work. For everything you need to know about losing weight and keeping it off FOR GOOD, you've got to read this book!"
*Kensley Palmer—CFL Running Back—Professional Fitness Trainer, Palmer's Pro Fitness*

"I lost 10 pounds in a month and gained lots of energy. I recommend this BootCamp to all of my friends who want quick results in a healthy way...two thumbs up!"
*BootCamper Denise Sabadel, Milan, Italy*

"For once, a FAST plan which is not a fad and which is healthy. I lost eight pounds and am still losing more because of all the new healthy habits I have integrated into my life. Thank you Valerie."
*BootCamper Edward Simson, New York, NY*

"**Valerie offers everyday life tips and tricks to help you lose weight and get fit in no time and in a healthy way. I highly recommend her book to anyone who wants to shed those extra pounds and develop healthy habits for a lifetime.**"
*Samuel Lebaron, Ph.D., MD—Director, Center for Education in Family and Community Medicine, Stanford School of Medicine*

"**This is a terrific program that taught me how to manage my eating and exercise in a time efficient manner. I had tried several quick fixes before but this one is the WINNER!**"
*BootCamper Roberta Amos, Calgary, AB*

# FOREWORD

**Steve Kemp**
**Olympic Decathlete**
**World Champion, Track and Field Athlete**

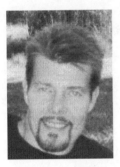

If you think about the times in your life when you had a burning desire to achieve a goal, it always began with visualizing the intended outcome. That's the best way to begin any journey. However, a vision without a great plan often causes the dream to end abruptly.

Valerie Orsoni-Vauthey's book, *30day BootCamp: Your Ultimate Weight Loss Plan* $^{TM}$, empowers people to turn their wishes and hopes for a healthy, fulfilling life into reality, by helping them understand that once they "know the path" and then "walk the path," they can actually "stay on the path" for their lifetime.

It is likely that each person reading this book has read or heard of any of the thousands of diet and nutrition books available on the market. This book is different than most, because it offers a foolproof way to achieve long-term success—which is what we all really want.

I believe we all want to look into the mirror—not only a few months from now, but five to ten years from now—and feel good about what we see. We want to feel healthy and energetic so that we can keep up with the adventure called "life" and stick around for our kids, the important relationships in our lives, our careers and, of course, for ourselves.

Your daily habits create your lifestyle. If you are operating on all cylinders, and your life and your health are where you want them to be, it is likely because of the habits you maintain. Conversely, if you are not satisfied with your life or your lifestyle, it is important to notice that your habits are creating that lifestyle, too. This book helps you redefine your lifestyle and create healthy lifestyle changes, one step at a time, so that you feel satisfied with your life in all areas.

In my experience as a Olympic decathlete and World Champion track and field athlete, I became aware that to get myself from point A (my dream) to point B (my goal), three elements were required: 1) knowledge of what it would take to become successful, 2) focus to carry out the plan that I created from the knowledge and 3) belief that I could do it.

You can think and achieve like a champion because Valerie has done the homework for you, and her insight and expertise will empower you through the knowledge contained in this book. It is easy to follow her simple principles, and develop supportive habits on a daily basis, because the book is so easy to read. It is one that you can easily pick up and refer to again and again. The constant support and friendly repetition keep you focused.

What I really like about Valerie's book is that it is not all about counting calories, getting obsessed about the latest fads, or going to the gym every day to exercise. It begins with simple adjustments in your daily habits. She teaches us that forming our healthiest habits can be fun and simple to apply. Because the two components of long-term success are healthy eating and moderate exercise, you will also learn the most effective exercises that you can do almost anywhere that both burn calories and tone your body at the same time. Many of these exercises are exactly the same ones I teach in my high-end, personal training classes. They are very effective for any age and for both women and men.

As you continue to lose weight, improve your health, de-stress, and increase your energy levels, your beliefs that YOU CAN DO IT are reinforced, giving you the mind-power you need for long-term success. You will finally achieve success in a program that you can—and will—stick to for the rest of your life!

Integrating the concepts and ideas of this book into your lifestyle will lead to simple, effective, and permanent weight loss, and lasting changes for a lifetime…guaranteed.

# From the author, with thanks...

**A thank-you note from Valerie Orsoni-Vauthey**

I would like to first thank my son, Baptiste, who is always my best supporter and who always believes in me even when I do not! Thank you to my beloved geek and to my dad for instilling in me this feeling that nothing is out of reach if I put my heart and soul to it (and some work of course!). Thanks to mom who always thinks that, whatever I do, I am the best person on earth and that I can only succeed.

Thanks to all of you who believed in this project: Annette Dykes, my 'coach' Rabbi Levin, Valerie Prigent, Michael Scadden, Sandra Harmon and Eva Ruimy—to name but a few.
Thank you to our "guinea pigs" who tried this bootcamp and shared their experience with me.
And, of course, thank you to those who did not believe in this project; your negative energy fueled my willingness to move forward at light speed.

And now, let's embark on our 30-day BootCamp! I guarantee you will enjoy this ride as much as I enjoyed writing it for YOU.

Love you all,
*Valerie*

# Introduction

**Congratulations on taking this healthy step to fast, effective and permanent weight loss!** I guarantee that by following my guidelines and suggestions, you WILL SEE RESULTS in less than 30 days. And if you continue using the guidelines and tips that you receive throughout this BootCamp, you will **keep the weight off PERMANENTLY**, because you will understand the key secrets of healthy nutrition and fitness. This program is a 30-day plan; but hopefully, most of what you learn you will take with you for the rest of your life.

**In order to lose weight, you need to be READY, really ready, to make some serious changes in your life.** Any program that promises quick-fix solutions to weight loss (lose 30 pounds in 30 days, for example) is preying on people's emotions. And most crash diets are extremely unhealthy in the long run, which is why I designed this program. I know that people want a quick solution to weight loss, so I'll give you one, in the healthiest possible way—no crazy metabolism boosting pills, no meal replacement bars or shakes, and most importantly, no counting!

You will need to eat healthy, nutritious foods, and get your body moving, every single day. I am not talking about hours sweating at the gym. The exercises you will perform while on this program can be done almost anywhere. The key here is to become more conscious of your daily level of activity. But I will talk about that in more detail a little later.

I understand that your life is dynamic, and that following a strict, regimented diet and exercise plan can be difficult for most people. Therefore, **much of this program is flexible, meaning that you can choose which breakfast, lunch or dinner you want to eat from the meal plans we provide.** Each meal ensures that you receive the nutrients you need to stay healthy over the next 30 days, while you continue to lose the extra weight for good.

**For the first week on the program, you will follow a regimented cleansing process** to prepare your body for healthy weight loss and to eliminate toxins in a healthy way. **The first week is non-alterable.** I strongly recommend that you follow my guidelines exactly. This BootCamp has been designed with you in mind—based on my extensive weight loss coaching experience. It has been proven time and time again to deliver results quickly and permanently. However, I am aware that some people have food allergies and/or specific medical conditions that require special attention. For those individual cases, I have created a "Substitutions Page" at the end of this introduction where you will find out how to swap certain items in the meal suggestions. If the exact product you are trying to avoid is not on the list, exercise your common sense, and make a choice that will serve you best. I believe that everyone can tap into what his or her body needs when one simply listens closely enough.

Remember, many crash diets have you eliminate entire food groups and/or count calories, fat grams and grams of protein to help you lose weight. But I don't believe in this kind of approach because I know counting ANYTHING results in obsessive-compulsive type behaviors (which, of course, are unhealthy). And that would defeat the purpose of "30-day BootCamp: Your Ultimate Weight Loss Plan." So, **NO COUNTING!** Simply follow these guidelines and listen to your body. Get to know what messages your body sends to you on a daily basis. You'll be surprised at what your body will tell you.

**You need to follow the meal suggestions, to the best of your ability, without alteration, so that each meal is rich in nutrients, which will keep your energy up and your level of satisfaction high.**

First things first, there are daily and weekly components to the program.

**DAILY KEY ELEMENTS:**

- **Daily Exercise Drills**—Exercises you can do almost ANYWHERE to tone and firm your muscles. You will also need to walk 30 minutes every day, on an empty stomach, throughout this program. PLUS get 60-minutes of cumulative exercise daily (more on this later).

- **Daily Nutritional Tips**—Tips and secrets to help you slim down and shape up. These educational tips will give you the inside scoops on why the foods you are eating are important to maintain a balanced diet.

- **Log:** At the end of each day you will fill in your log. First, make sure to put the date in the empty field, and then use the "smilies" to rate how you felt overall throughout the day, how you felt your diet was (did you follow the BootCamp seriously or not), how much exercise you did, and what your overall stress level was like. If you feel you did what the BootCamp suggested for that particular day—or even more—circle the ☺; if you believe you could have done more, circle the ☺ and if you did not do any-thing—which I do not recommend—circle the ☹.

After that, write down what you had for breakfast, lunch, and din-ner, and for any extra meal, if any. This will help you keep track of the invisible calories you may be ingesting (trying something new at the market, tasting while cooking, taking a cookie at work, etc…). Most people are surprised at first, when they realize that they eat more than they think.

Next, track your fluid intake. You know how important it is to keep your body hydrated so it's imperative that you log your daily fluid intake as well (preferably water or decaf tea).

Then, circle "yes" or "no" if you had transfats in your food (you will learn more about transfats in this BootCamp), refined carbs (white bread, cookies, white pasta, candies, etc…) and if you cooked your own food or if you bought it already made. This will help you make your own diagnosis as to what you can improve day after day.

Lastly, you will log your fitness activity for each day. Circle ☑ if you did something and ☒ if you did not do anything, in each cate-gory. Write the type of activity you did on the line provided (exam-ple: yoga for flexibility, Taebo™ for cardio, etc…) and for how long you exercised. Remember to include how many steps you walked. Check out the example of a daily log at the end of this introduction for guidance, if you need it.

## WEEKLY KEY ELEMENTS:

- **Healthy, Balanced Meal Plans**
- **Weekly Shopping Lists**
- **Weekly MetaBoost Cards**
- **Weekly Recipes**

The greatest part about this program is that its offers **recipes and meal plans for ALL preferences.** You will get vegan dishes, vegetarian dishes, light meals, party dishes, restaurant suggestions...everything you need to make your weight-loss journey as easy as possible. But remember: try to follow the meal plans to a tee for Week 1. After the Jump-Start Program (Days 3–7), with the exception of Day 15 and 16, you can mix and match meal plans for breakfast, lunch and dinner.

You may note that many of these recipes serve four or more people, yet this book is directed to one person: YOU. Is all the extra food to be thrown out? It certainly isn't supposed to be eaten by you, is it? Why aren't the recipes single servings?

The answer to these questions is simple: some of the recipes are single servings, while others are for more people because this is not a diet, and these recipes are not meant to exclude your family or friends from your healthy lifestyle.

It seems like a lot to remember, but don't worry...you will get reminders and tips along the way.

I have also created a list of "healthier" fast-food choices. (You will get this list at the beginning of Week 2.) If you are too busy to prepare your meals—and I know that this sometimes happens—you can use the list as a reference to help you make healthier choices at the drive-thru window. But, if at all possible, follow the main meal suggestions first and only go to the drive-thru as a last resort.

Each day includes one page of the **"Ultimate Daily Fitness and Diet Log,"** which will make your weight-loss journey easy to track. I strongly suggest you download a full, printable copy, so that you have it on hand at all times (and you can keep your book in mint condition.)

You can download your full, FREE copy by going to:
www.MyPrivateCoach.com/bootcamp_log

Username: superreader—Password: icandothis

# YOU CAN DO THIS!

First, **BEGIN THIS PROGRAM ON A SATURDAY**. Why? There are two cleanses that require juicing and the recipes are more difficult to prepare if you are out of your home. So, by starting on a Saturday, both cleanse days will take place on Sundays. PLUS, on a cleanse day, you may have less energy than normal, so I recommend doing the cleanses on a day off. If today is any other day than Saturday, GET READY by completing the following SEVEN steps:

1. **Go Grocery Shopping.** Buy everything you need from your Week 1 Shopping List.

2. **Eliminate Temptations.** Throw away all high-sugar, high-fat foods in your fridge and home.

3. **Purchase your "Equipment."** In order to participate fully in this BootCamp, you will need a juicer, a pedometer, and a pair of sneakers. I have searched high and low for the best products for your weight-loss journey. My top picks are: the Breville Juice Fountain, the FM Pedometer, the Nike Women's Shox TL or Nike Women's Air Alvord 2, and the Nike Men's Air Zoom Swift Vapor Trainer. These are the highest quality products I have found on the market at a very reasonable price.

   I know you're busy, so I have created an online store for your convenience. If you don't have time to shop for these products on your own, feel free to visit the MyPrivateCoach website to buy what you need.

   **Go to: http://www.MyPrivateCoach.com/store
   and order your products before we begin.**

4. **Walk.** Begin walking for 30 minutes every morning after drinking one glass of water or green tea (do not consume anything else).

You will do this every morning throughout the BootCamp. Pick up the pace and get your heart pumping!

5. **Detox.** Avoid red meats, high-sugar foods, and high-fat dairy products (the low-fat versions are okay, but if you can, choose dairy alternatives like soy, rice or almond milk and yogurt instead of dairy products).

6. **Drink Water.** Make sure you drink AT LEAST eight glasses of water per day while on this program. (Side note: Keep in mind that different people have different needs. Some people only need six glasses of water per day, while others need 12 or more. The best way to tell if you are dehydrated is to look at the color of your urine. If it is very dark, then you need more water. If it is clear, you're on the right track.)

7. **Weigh-In.** Weigh yourself on Day 1 to determine your starting point and input your result in the "Ultimate Daily Fitness and Diet Log." We will do a weigh-in every week to track your progress.

ഇ

### Creating the Camp...

As you dive into this BootCamp with me you may begin to wonder things like:

*Why on earth do we start with a cleansing day?*
*Why is week 1 so strict?*
*Why do we have another cleansing day on Day 15?*
*Why do we keep adding exercises as the BootCamp progresses?*
*etc......*

The fact that you are wondering is actually great news, because it shows that you like to *think* about a program before diving in whole-heartedly, and because of this, you will likely learn a lot from this program and will take these tips and tricks with you to use for the rest of your life. Good for you!

So, let us unravel the mystery behind the creation of this BootCamp...

Week 1 is the strictest week, because empirically the coaches at MyPrivateCoach have noticed that 100% of our BootCampers always had the highest level of motivation during the first week. So I want you to make the most out of it! This week is also important from a cleansing perspective. Once you are on track, I help you make smart choices as we proceed, but you won't do a "week 1" again. Promise. After this regimented week, I bring back freedom of choice when it comes to meals, which is what makes this BootCamp different than any other, and also why It works long-term.

You will also notice that as the BootCamp progresses, we continue to ramp up the fitness component of the program. Why? Because as you start shedding pounds, you will be more and more motivated to hit the trails, do a MetaBoost workout or simply walk around your neighborhood. I also assume that not all of us are used to exercising every day, so I opted for a crescendo approach: start slowly and gradually increase the intensity and frequency of your fitness sessions.

The cleansing days serve two purposes:

1. Cleansing on the first day of the BootCamp will help you eliminate unwanted toxins, and will get you started truly because it takes discipline and you will subconsciously recognize that you are doing yourself good. This greatly increases self-esteem, and will help you stay focused on the first week. Guaranteed!
2. Cleansing at mid-BootCamp will make sure you stay on track, stay focused and will eliminate even further toxins.

One other important aspect of the cleansing process, by eating no solid foods, is that it helps you become more aware of what true hunger really feels like; therefore, you will get in better touch with your body's signals for hunger and satiety. This is a critical aspect of our approach: knowing when your body requires food, not when your mind "thinks" you're hungry.

Now that my secrets are out, it's time to BEGIN…

## EXAMPLE
### Daily Fitness & Diet Log

Date **05/1/06**

Overall Feeling Today:
Overall Diet:

Overall Fitness:
Overall Stress Level:

### Diet...

| Breakfast | Lunch | Dinner |
|---|---|---|
| 2 slice bread | 1 apple | 1 bowl soup |
| 1 avocado | Tomato Soup | 1 plain yogurt |
| 1 cup blueberies | | a few berries |
| 1 decaf tea | | Stevia |

Extra meal (if any): **1 apple @ 4 pm**

Fluid Intake: **9** cups. Type of fluid: **WATER**

Transfat?... yes /(no)    Refined carbs?... yes /(no)    Home-made food?.. (yes) no

### Fitness...

How many steps: **12,000**

| | | |
|---|---|---|
| Flexibility | ☑: **YOGA** | ⏱: **15 min** |
| MetaBoost | ☑: **# 2** | ⏱: **10 min** |
| Strength | ☑ | ⏱ |
| Cardio | ☑: **TAEBO** | ⏱: **45** |
| Other | ☑ | ⏱ |

# ಐ **Substitutions** ಐ

For those of us who have a known allergy to specific foods, a medical condition or a special diet I have created this list of possible swaps:

**Yeast**: Select yeast-free whole wheat bread (I love the Mana Brand from Nature's Path).

**Milk:** Can easily be replaced by soymilk or, even better, by home-made almond milk: soak 1 cup of almonds overnight and blend with 2 cups of water. Drain through a mesh filter. Add 2 tablespoons raw agave nectar and 1 teaspoon vanilla extract. For a great shake add a banana and a few berries and blend.

**Eggs:** Eggs can be replaced by egg substitutes (usually found in natural food stores) or for baking:

- 1 tsp. baking powder, 1 T. liquid, 1 T. vinegar or
- 1 tsp. yeast dissolved in 1/4 cup warm water or
- 1 1/2 T. water, 1 1/2 T. oil, 1 tsp. baking powder or
- 1 packet gelatin, 2 T. warm water. Do not mix until ready to use.

**Peanuts/Nuts:** Since most experts recommend that peanut-allergic patients avoid tree nuts as well, stay away from all nuts if you think you may develop an allergic reaction. You can replace nuts by seeds: sunflower seeds and pumpkin seeds are a good alternative. If you love peanut butter (I personally love raw almond butter) you can get almost the same taste sensation with raw pumpkin seed butter.

**Fish/Shellfish:** Replace by tofu if you are vegetarian or by grilled chicken if you like animal protein. A plain yogurt can do the trick too from a protein perspective. You can also substitute one egg for one serving of fish.

**Soy**: Soybeans can be found in thousands of processed foods, so make sure you check the labels before buying vegetarian, ready-made foods. Soymilk can be replaced by regular milk (or almond milk—my favorite). Soybeans or edamame can be replaced by fresh sweet peas. Lean meat or fish can replace tofu if you are not vegetarian. If you are vegan/vegetarian and wish to eat something with some consistency, you can go for pates and patties made of sunflower seeds, soaked almonds, and sprouted grains. You can find those recipes in several books geared towards food allergies and/or recipe books for raw-foodists.

**Wheat**: Can be replaced by corn flour, rice flour and potato starch; usually a combination of these three works best.

**Berries**: You can replace berries in your cleansing drinks or smoothies by any other dark-colored fruit: very ripe apricots, cherries, or nectarines, for example.

**Meat/Fish/Dairy:** If you are vegan you can replace all animal protein sources by nuts, sprouted grains and/or tofu.

# Day 1: Let's Get Started!

Remember to begin Day 1 on a Saturday. Are you ready to get started? Yes? PERFECT. You should now have everything you need for this program.

To get started, make sure you weigh yourself so that you know your starting point, and record your weight in your logbook. If you can, use a scale that calculates your body fat percentage. My favorite is the Tanita Family Model Scale, which is also available at the MyPrivateCoach. com store (http://www.MyPrivateCoach.com/store).

Here are the average body fat categories[*] for men and women:

| Classification | Women—%fat | Men—%fat |
|---|---|---|
| Essential Fat | 10–12% | 2–4% |
| Athlete | 14–20% | 6–13% |
| Fitness | 21–24% | 14–17% |
| Acceptable | 25–31% | 18–25% |
| Obese | 32% + | 25% + |

* American Council on Exercise

To be healthy, you should aim for a body fat % in the athlete, fitness or lower range of the acceptable category.

**Today's Goodies:**

- Day 1 Meal Plan
- Week 1 Shopping List
- Tomato Soup with Edamame Recipe
- Daily Fitness & Diet Log

**Remember, you MUST follow all guidelines for Week 1 without making any changes or alterations (unless you have a specific medical condition).**

Be sure to follow all nutritional guidelines for today (Day 1).

## EXERCISE DRILL—Day 1—WALK, WALK, WALK

Your assignment for the next 30 days is to walk for 30 minutes, every morning, on an empty stomach. Make sure you drink one glass of water first. If you absolutely cannot walk for 30 minutes in the morning, then make sure you walk 30 minutes at another time of day, and make sure it is on an EMPTY STOMACH (before lunch or dinner).

Several studies have shown that **when you exercise on an empty stomach, YOU WILL LOSE WEIGHT** because you will tap into your fat stores for the energy you need to contract your muscles, rather than using the energy (glucose) that is in your bloodstream, which tends to be used first when you exercise after you eat.

## NUTRITIONAL TIP—Day 1

In preparation for the 3-Color Cleanse™ tomorrow, it is critical that you eat mainly fruits, vegetables, soups, plain yogurt, and low glycemic index carbohydrates (like chick peas, slow-cooked oatmeal, or whole-wheat pasta, for example) today. If you eat foods high in fat and protein, your body is more likely to feel deprived tomorrow, and it will be difficult to stick to the 3-Color Cleanse™. The 3-Color Cleanse™ is the trademark of "30-day BootCamp: Your Ultimate Weight Loss Plan," so set yourself up to win.

Remember, **you will need a juicer tomorrow and on Day 16**, and for several other recipes that are included with this program. If you do not have a juicer yet, you can go to a juice bar tomorrow and request the specific ingredients listed in your meal plan for your breakfast, lunch and dinner, but this will be more expensive in the long run. I highly recommend the Breville Juice Fountain because it is extremely user-friendly, makes delicious juices, and is so easy to clean.

See you tomorrow,

*Valerie Your Private Coach*

# Meal Suggestions—Day 1—Light

## 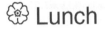 Breakfast

2 slices whole-grain bread ~~w/PB~~
~~1 avocado~~
1 cup strawberries

## 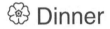 Lunch

1 apple
**\*Tomato Soup with Edamame\***

## Dinner

1 bowl light soup
1 plain yogurt
Stevia

# ഔ Shopping List—Week 1 ഔ

## Vegetables, Legumes & Nuts

- 1 bunch of collard leaves (or a bunch of spinach)
- 1 celery stalk
- 1 carrot
- 1 fresh ginger slice
- 2 baby carrots
- 2 cans of soup (precooked, light type)
- Arugula salad
- 1 pound salad mix
- 2 fresh bunches of spinach
- 6 cups button mushrooms
- Hazelnuts
- 2 falafels
- 2 cans of organic, cooked garbanzo beans
- 1 can pinto beans
- 1 can black beans
- 1 head of garlic
- 4 ripe tomatoes
- Fresh oregano
- Fresh cilantro (optional)
- 2 shallots
- 3 eggplants

## Fruit

- 10 apples
- 1 cup dried apple rings
- 3 pounds strawberries
- ½ cup dried strawberries
- 3 oranges
- 1 cup blueberries (wild is better)
- ½ cup blackberries (can be replaced with more blueberries)
- 1 cup raspberries
- 1 avocado
- 1 cup raisins
- 1 cup dried apricots
- 3 lemons
- 1 grapefruit
- 1 lime
- 1 honeydew melon
- 1 ripe avocado
- Strawberry preserve

## Eggs & Dairy

- 4 plain yogurt
- 1 Greek yogurt
- Fresh mozzarella
- Low-fat cottage cheese
- 1 cup shredded low-fat cheddar cheese

## Meat, Fish & Tofu

- 1 slice of cold turkey
- 1 pound fresh, wild shrimp
- 1 veggie burger
- 1 turkey patty
- Small package of smoked wild salmon
- Anchovy filet (optional)
- 1 small can of tuna in water (no salt added)
- 1 large can of tuna
- Gardenburger meatless riblets

| Oils & Sweets | Miscellaneous |
|---|---|
| - Olive oil<br>- Canola oil<br>- Canola oil spray | - Green tea<br>- Decaf black tea<br>- Black tea<br>- Chamomile tea<br>- 7 slices whole-grain bread<br>- 2 whole-wheat pita bread<br>- Sprouted grain tortillas (Ezekiel brand)<br>- Tahini paste (sesame)<br>- Stevia<br>- Balsamic vinegar<br>- Sea salt<br>- Soyonnaise<br>- Cumin<br>- Curry<br>- Onion powder<br>- Slow-cooked oatmeal<br>- Dijon mustard<br>- 1 can low-fat coconut milk<br>- Low-sodium soy sauce<br>- 1 packet of instant miso soup |

## Tomato Soup with Edamame

**You can make this colorful soup in the blink of an eye; it provides healthy fiber and the highest possible level of cancer-fighting lycopene.**

### Ingredients:

- 2 cups of tomato soup (preferably fresh and organic, but from a can will work as well)
- Frozen or fresh edamame (soybeans, shelled)
- Oregano

### Directions:

**-1-** Heat tomato soup until serving temperature is reached (140 to 150 degrees).
**-2-** Warm up edamame beans.
**-3-** Pour tomato soup in a bowl.
**-4-** Sprinkle approx. 20 edamame beans.
**-5-** Sprinkle oregano.

Enjoy!

Serves 1

### Variations:

If you don't have edamame, fava beans will work fine, as will peas.

# Daily Fitness & Diet Log

Date [            ]                                Weight [            ]

Overall Feeling Today:   ☺ ☺ ☹         Overall Fitness:        ☺ ☺ ☹
Overall Diet:            ☺ ☺ ☹         Overall Stress Level:   ☺ ☺ ☹

## Diet...

| Breakfast | Lunch | Dinner |
| --- | --- | --- |
| _____ | _____ | _____ |
| _____ | _____ | _____ |
| _____ | _____ | _____ |
| _____ | _____ | _____ |
| _____ | _____ | _____ |

Extra meal (if any): _____

Fluid Intake: [            ] cups. Type of fluid: _____

Trans fats?... yes / no     Refined carbs?... yes / no     Home-made food?... yes / no

## Fitness...                     How many steps: [            ]

Flexibility     ☑☒: _____     🕐: _____

MetaBoost       ☑☒: _____     🕐: _____

Strength        ☑☒: _____     🕐: _____

Cardio          ☑☒: _____     🕐: _____

Other           ☑☒: _____     🕐: _____

# Day 2: 3-Color Cleanse™

**It's 3-Color Cleanse™ Day!**

Remember, **you will need your juicer today.** If you do not have a juicer yet, you can order your juices at a juice bar for breakfast, lunch and dinner. This will be more expensive in the long run, but it is certainly an option. You will be receiving several other juice recipes throughout this BootCamp, so having your own juicer will give you the flexibility of creating your juices from home. Besides, having your own juicer will give you the joy of creating your own recipes at the end of this program. (See the benefits of juicing below…)

**Today, you will eat no solid foods.** You will have your Green Boost in the morning, the Orange Boost in the afternoon, and the Blue Boost in the evening. In between juices, you may drink as much green tea or regular tea as you wish (caffeinated or decaf are fine—you choose).

**Today's Goodies:**

- Day 2 Meal Plan
- Morning Green Boost Recipe
- Orange Boost Recipe
- Blue Boost Recipe
- Daily Fitness & Diet Log

## EXERCISE DRILL—Day 2—An Easy Day…

Because you will be consuming fewer calories today, make today an easy day as far as exercise.

It is beneficial that you still take your 30-minute walk this morning, but don't push yourself too much. Choose activities today that require less physical energy (reading, writing, arts, music—even paperwork if it needs to be done—etc.). Trust me, there will be plenty of exercise to be done over the next 28 days.

## NUTRITIONAL TIP—Day 2

**Fruits and vegetables provide vitamins, minerals, essential fatty acids, carbohydrates, and proteins that are vital for good health.** Although eating fruits and vegetables in their natural state does provide a substantial amount of vitamins and minerals, juicing can help us obtain the maximum benefits of these micronutrients because it is easier to consume the juice of five carrots, than it is to eat five carrots whole.

When we juice our fruits and vegetables, we are **able to absorb these nutrients more quickly into the bloodstream, in a highly condensed form** (kind of like a multivitamin, but with the benefits of live food). Fiber is essential to health, so be sure to continue eating raw fruits, vegetables, legumes and whole grains, along with fresh juices, to gain the maximum amount of nutritional value from your diet. But a day without fiber is absolutely okay.

You will find that when you make juicing a part of your daily diet, you gain increased energy, a glowing complexion, a strengthened immune system, stronger bones, and you reduce your risk for disease. I recommend that you drink at least 16 ounces of freshly squeezed juice each day.

You're on track now…

See you tomorrow,

*Valerie Your Private Coach*

# Meal Suggestions—Day 2
# 3-Color Cleanse™

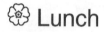 ## Breakfast

1 cup of Green Tea
**\*1 8-oz. glass Morning Green Boost\***

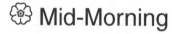 ## Mid-Morning

1 cup of Black Tea

## Lunch

1 cup of Green Tea
**\*1 8-oz. glass of Orange Boost\***

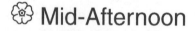 ## Mid-Afternoon

1 cup of Decaf Black Tea

## Dinner

1 cup of Decaf Green Tea
**\*1 8-oz. glass of Blue Smoothing Boost\***

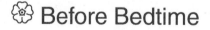 ## Before Bedtime

1 cup of Chamomile Tea

# Morning Green Boost

. For this drink, you will need a juicer. The search for a juicer took me several months, as so many I tried leaked and could not handle more than one juicing without needing to be cleaned, etc...I finally settled on a Breville Juicer (you can put a whole apple directly in the feeder).

. The Morning Green Boost provides several much-needed nutrients and phytochemicals including:

. You will get **your daily vitamin C** recommended by the FDA, thanks to the apple and celery.

. You will get **calcium from the collard leaves**.

. You will get **vitamin A from the carrot.**

. In addition to this impressive list, **celery also provides 15% of your daily potassium** requirements.

## Ingredients:

- 1 apple
- 1 collard leaf (or half a bunch of spinach)
- 1 stalk of celery
- 4 strawberries
- 1 carrot
- 1 fresh ginger slice

## Directions:

**-1-** Rinse and pat dry all fruits/veggies. You can put your fruits/veggies directly in the juicer—no need to peel (except ginger root).

**-2-** Juice and drink right away as antioxidants lose their potency as time passes.

Enjoy!

&

# Orange Boost

. For this drink, you will need your juicer.
. The Orange Boost will provide plenty of the much-needed nutrients and phyto-chemicals you need daily.
. **You will get your daily Vitamin C recommended by the FDA, thanks to the apple and orange, and Vitamin A from the carrots ("carotene") and the straw-berries.**

## Ingredients:

- 1 apple
- 1 orange
- 2 baby carrots
- 3 strawberries

## Directions:

**-1-** Rinse and pat dry all fruits/veggies. You can put your fruits/veggies directly in the juicer—no need to peel.
**-2-** Juice and drink right away as antioxidants lose their potency as time passes.

Enjoy!

୫ଠ

# Blue Smoothing Boost

. For this drink, you will need your juicer.

. The Blue Smoothing Boost will provide plenty of the much-needed nutrients and phytochemicals you need daily.

. **You will get your daily vitamin C recommended by the FDA, thanks to the apple, and vitamin A from the strawberries ("carotene").**

. Just one serving of blueberries provides as many antioxidants as five servings of carrots, apples, broccoli or squash.

. **In fact, USDA studies rank blueberries number one in antioxidant activity compared with 40 other fruits and vegetables.**

. Blueberries are particularly high in flavonoid anthocyanin (a potent antioxidant), which is concentrated in the skin and gives blueberries their intense blue-purple color. This natural compound is linked with many health benefits, including reducing eyestrain and improving night vision.

## Ingredients:

- 1 cup blueberries (wild is better)
- 5 strawberries
- 1 apple
- ½ cup blackberries (can be replaced with more blueberries)

## Directions:

**-1-** Rinse and pat dry all fruits/veggies. You can put your fruits/veggies directly in the juicer—no need to peel.

**-2-** Juice and drink right away as antioxidants lose their potency as time passes.

Enjoy!

&

# Daily Fitness & Diet Log

Date [          ]

Overall Feeling Today: ☺ ☺ ☹          Overall Fitness:          ☺ ☺ ☹
Overall Diet: ☺ ☺ ☹                   Overall Stress Level:    ☺ ☺ ☹

## Diet...

| Breakfast | Lunch | Dinner |
| --- | --- | --- |
| _____ | _____ | _____ |
| _____ | _____ | _____ |
| _____ | _____ | _____ |
| _____ | _____ | _____ |
| _____ | _____ | _____ |

Extra meal (if any): _____

Fluid Intake: [          ] cups. Type of fluid: _____

Trans fats?... yes / no          Refined carbs?... yes / no          Home-made food?... yes / no

## Fitness...          How many steps: [          ]

Flexibility      ☑☒: _____      ①: _____

MetaBoost       ☑☒: _____      ①: _____

Strength        ☑☒: _____      ①: _____

Cardio          ☑☒: _____      ①: _____

Other           ☑☒: _____      ①: _____

# Day 3: Jump-Start (Days 3–7)

**Now we're on to the Jump-Start Program!**

Remember, **the next five days must be followed without alteration.** Today, we'll start with the Green Boost again, as well as a few other solid foods, to make this breakfast more nutritionally complete. Lunch and dinner are also light, but they are very balanced and provide the vitamins and minerals you need for proper physiological function.

You may sip on decaf teas throughout the day to ease hunger. Filling yourself up with liquids will send the "full" signal to your brain, so always reach for water or tea before you opt for a snack or meal. Besides, 80% of the time that you feel hungry, you are actually thirsty. So drink up!

Also, remember to log your progress in your **"Ultimate Daily Fitness and Diet Log"**.

**Today's Goodies:**

- Day 3 Meal Plan
- Homemade Hummus Recipe
- Tomato Mozzarella Salad Recipe
- Daily Fitness & Diet Log

## EXERCISE DRILL—Day 3—10,000 Steps a Day

In addition to your daily 30-minute walk on an empty stomach, you also need an average of 60 minutes of accumulated exercise per day (based on the Surgeon General's recommendations). Each 15-minute period counts towards the 60-minute goal.

This is where your pedometer comes in handy. Sixty minutes of accumulated activity plus your 30-minute daily walk will add up to approximately 10,000 steps per day (or more). A pedometer will help you track your steps.

You will need to find four 15-minute intervals SOMEWHERE throughout your day to walk, walk, walk! You can wake up a bit earlier, walk during your lunch hour or after dinner, or park further away from work and walk 30 minutes to and from your office, etc…even walking around the grocery store counts. Just MOVE!

If you already have an active lifestyle, then pick things up a notch by either increasing the speed, duration or frequency of your exercise. This will challenge your body in new ways if you have reached a plateau.

***Another tip:*** If you know ahead of time that it will be difficult to find 60-minutes of free time to move your body today (or any day of this program), go out for a 5- to 10-minute walk every two hours. This counts towards your 60-minute daily goal. If you have to make phone calls, take your cell phone and walk while you talk instead of staying at your desk.

But remember, the 30-minute daily walk on an empty stomach must be done all at once (preferably in the morning).

## NUTRITIONAL TIP—Day 3—Eat Your Tomatoes

Tomatoes contain large amounts of vitamin C, vitamin A, potassium and iron.

The red pigment found in tomatoes is called lycopene. This compound acts as an antioxidant, neutralizing free radicals that can damage cells in the body.

An interesting fact about tomatoes is that cooked tomatoes actually contain MORE lycopene than raw tomatoes. This is interesting since heat usually alters the nutrient value of foods in a negative way. But tomatoes are different. And studies have shown that men and women who eat up to 10 servings of tomatoes per week can reduce their risk of cancer by up to 45%.

Be Strong!

## *Valerie Your Private Coach*

P.S. Did you remember your 30-minute walk this morning?

# Meal Suggestions—Day 3

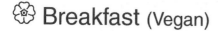 ## Breakfast (Vegan)

**\*Morning Green Boost\***
1 cup Greek yogurt (or soy yogurt)
¼ cup hazelnuts
¼ cup dried apricots
Stevia

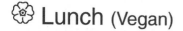 ## Lunch (Vegan)

1 whole-wheat pita bread
**\*Hummus\***
2 falafels
1 apple

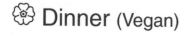 ## Dinner (Vegan)

**\*Tomato Mozzarella salad\***
1 slice of turkey
1 yogurt
1 apple

# Hummus

This is a tasty and very healthy **dip, side dish and spread** that I recommend you always keep ready in your fridge to satisfy your cravings for salt or carbs.

## Ingredients:

1 can of organic, cooked garbanzo beans
½ lemon (juice)
⅓ cup of olive oil (virgin, first cold press)
½ teaspoon of tahini paste (sesame paste)
1 clove of garlic
Salt to taste

## Directions:

Put all ingredients in a mixer/blender until you get a smooth puree. Some people prefer it coarse. It is up to you.

## Variations:

You can vary the taste by doing the following:

Adding 2 teaspoons of cumin
Or
Adding 2 teaspoons of paprika
Or
No tahini (sesame paste)
Or
Adding 1 cup of fresh white mushrooms
Or
Be creative!

## Serving suggestions:

Put the mixture in a serving bowl; pour some olive oil on top and a few olives for visual appeal.

℘

# Tomato Mozzarella Salad

**This easy, Mediterranean salad is loaded with muscle-building proteins and the highest possible level of lycopene, an antioxidant present in tomatoes that has been linked to reduced cancer rates.**

*Antioxidants help counteract the harmful effects of substances called "free radicals," which are thought to contribute to many chronic diseases and age-related processes in the body.*

## Ingredients:

- Ripe tomatoes (preferably organic)
- Fresh mozzarella
- Olive oil
- Oregano
- Salt to taste

## Directions:

-1- Slice tomatoes. Slice mozzarella.
-2- Arrange them on a plate, putting one slice of mozzarella over a slice of tomato, exposing half an inch of the lower slice. Continue until you have used all the slices.
-3- Drizzle a little bit of olive oil on top.
-4- Sprinkle oregano and salt to taste.

Enjoy!

૪૭

# Daily Fitness & Diet Log

Date [                    ]

| | | | |
|---|---|---|---|
| Overall Feeling Today: | ☺ ☺ ☹ | Overall Fitness: | ☺ ☺ ☹ |
| Overall Diet: | ☺ ☺ ☹ | Overall Stress Level: | ☺ ☺ ☹ |

## Diet...

| Breakfast | Lunch | Dinner |
|---|---|---|
| _____ | _____ | _____ |
| _____ | _____ | _____ |
| _____ | _____ | _____ |
| _____ | _____ | _____ |
| _____ | _____ | _____ |

Extra meal (if any): _____

Fluid Intake: [          ] cups. Type of fluid: _____

Trans fats?... yes / no      Refined carbs?... yes / no      Home-made food?... yes / no

## Fitness...

How many steps: [          ]

| | | |
|---|---|---|
| Flexibility | ☑☒: _____ | ⏱: _____ |
| MetaBoost | ☑☒: _____ | ⏱: _____ |
| Strength | ☑☒: _____ | ⏱: _____ |
| Cardio | ☑☒: _____ | ⏱: _____ |
| Other | ☑☒: _____ | ⏱: _____ |

# Day 4: Jump-Start (Days 3–7)

**You're doing GREAT!**

**Three days down, only 27 more to go.** How are you feeling today? One of the greatest sources of motivation is to know your "why." Why do you want to lose weight? What will you accomplish by losing weight healthfully? How will you feel once you have lost those extra pounds?

**When you have a reason to do something, you will be more compelled to follow through with your commitment.** Jim Rohn, a motivational speaker and trainer says, "The bigger the 'why,' the easier the 'how.'"

So what is your "why"? Ask yourself why you want to lose weight and imagine how you will feel when you do. Feel it deep within you, and tap into that feeling whenever you feel like quitting. When you know your "why," the "how" becomes rather simple.

I guarantee that there will be moments when you feel like throwing in the towel; but **when you keep your "why" in the forefront of your mind, nothing will stand in your way!**

**Today's Goodies:**

- Day 4 Meal Plan
- Grilled Shrimp Recipe
- Spinach Strawberry Apple Salad Recipe
- Daily Fitness & Diet Log

## EXERCISE DRILL—Day 4—Strong Arms

The following exercise will help you to easily tone the backs of your upper arms (triceps). As soon as you read this, and several times today (at least each time you go to the restroom), stand straight in front of a wall with your arms straight at eye level. Place your palms on the wall and do 20 standing push-ups. With each push-up, push your body away from the wall a little bit harder.

Aim for 50 reps, and repeat throughout the day. You really can do this exercise anywhere. You can even exercise against your car in a parking lot if you want to.

To increase the difficulty of this exercise, rotate your hands inwards so that your fingers touch...and remember to stretch when you're done. The best way to stretch your triceps is to lift one arm overhead and bend at the elbow so that your hand is behind your head. With the other arm, push down on the elbow until you feel a stretch in your bent arm. Hold the stretch for 20 seconds. Repeat with the other arm.

Getting stronger day by day...

## NUTRITIONAL TIP—Day 4

In the past, shellfish were excluded from low-cholesterol diets because they were thought to be high in cholesterol. However, new, sophisticated measuring techniques proved that cholesterol levels of many shellfish are much lower than was previously believed.

In fact, **shrimp was found to have a large percentage of non-cholesterol sterols that appear to have a positive effect on cholesterol levels. The sterols actually inhibit the absorption of cholesterol eaten at the same meal.** Cholesterol levels in crustaceans such as crab and lobster are similar to that found in the dark meat of chicken.

While the cholesterol levels in shrimp vary considerably by species, levels are generally 1½ to 2 times higher than in the dark meat of chicken, but far less than the cholesterol level in eggs.

Therefore, because shellfish contain very little saturated fat, they are no longer excluded from typical, low-cholesterol diets.

See you tomorrow,

*Valerie Your Private Coach*

# Meal Suggestions—Day 4

## ✤ Breakfast (Vegan)

Slow-cooked oatmeal
1 grapefruit
Stevia

## ✤ Lunch (Light)

Salad mix + 3 tablespoons vinaigrette
**\*Grilled Shrimp\***
1 apple

## ✤ Dinner

**\*Spinach Strawberry Apple Salad\***
Grilled turkey patty
1 plain yogurt
Stevia

# Grilled Shrimp

. Shrimp contains a large percentage of non-cholesterol sterols which **inhibit the absorption of cholesterol eaten at the same meal.**
. While the cholesterol in shrimp varies considerably by species, it generally is 1½ times higher than in the dark meat of chicken, but far less than in eggs. So, because shellfish contain very little saturated fat, they are no longer excluded from typical, low-cholesterol diets.

## Ingredients:

- 1 pound fresh wild shrimp (avoid farm-raised shrimp, which contain a high level of pollutants and saturated fat because of their diet and lack of exercise)
- Canola oil spray
- Thyme (to taste)
- The juice of one lime per person
- Low-fat coconut milk (1 small can)
- Curry

## Directions:

-1- Preheat skillet and spray canola oil.
-2- When the skillet is hot, sauté the shrimp until well cooked.
-3- Add lime juice, salt (if needed) and coconut milk.
-4- Sprinkle curry.

Enjoy right away, as this dish is not intended to be reheated.

Serves 2.

&

# Spinach Strawberry Apple Salad

Spinach! This nutrient-rich, dark, leafy green provide calcium, magnesium, vitamin B6 and several other phytochemicals that are still being studied for their cancer-fighting capabilities.
. Vitamin B6 is indispensable for your body to be able to process magnesium. A lack of magnesium may lead to noise sensitivities, nervousness, Irritability, mental depression, confusion, twitching, trembling, apprehension, insomnia, muscle weakness and cramps in the toes, feet, legs, or fingers.

## Ingredients:

- 2 fresh bunches of spinach, rinsed, drained, and pat-dried
- ½ cup dried strawberries, sliced
- 1 cup of dried apple rings or half slices
- 2 tablespoons canola oil
- 1 tablespoon balsamic vinegar
- 1 teaspoon Dijon mustard
- 1 tablespoon minced shallots
- Salt and pepper to taste

## Directions:

-1- Prepare vinaigrette by mixing oil, vinegar, Dijon mustard and shallots in a small bowl.
-2- Put spinach in a large salad bowl. Add all but one tablespoon of vinaigrette.
-3- Top with dried strawberries and dried apples and drizzle remaining dressing on top.

Serves 4.

Enjoy!

## Variations:

As a blue cheese lover, I added blue cheese to this salad and it was delicious (but just a tiny bit ☺

# Daily Fitness & Diet Log

Date [                    ]

| | | | |
|---|---|---|---|
| Overall Feeling Today: | ☺ ☺ ☹ | Overall Fitness: | ☺ ☺ ☹ |
| Overall Diet: | ☺ ☺ ☹ | Overall Stress Level: | ☺ ☺ ☹ |

## Diet...

| Breakfast | Lunch | Dinner |
|---|---|---|
| _____ | _____ | _____ |
| _____ | _____ | _____ |
| _____ | _____ | _____ |
| _____ | _____ | _____ |
| _____ | _____ | _____ |

Extra meal (if any): _____

Fluid Intake: [            ] cups. Type of fluid: _____

Trans fats?... yes / no    Refined carbs?... yes / no    Home-made food?... yes / no

## Fitness...

How many steps: [            ]

| | | |
|---|---|---|
| Flexibility | ☑☒: _____ | ⏱: _____ |
| MetaBoost | ☑☒: _____ | ⏱: _____ |
| Strength | ☑☒: _____ | ⏱: _____ |
| Cardio | ☑☒: _____ | ⏱: _____ |
| Other | ☑☒: _____ | ⏱: _____ |

# Day 5: Jump-Start (Days 3–7)

**You are making tremendous progress!**

Every day, you are getting closer and closer to your goal: to lose weight, increase your energy, and feel better all around. That should be motivation enough to keep going!

But if you're having a hard time staying away from snacks, especially late at night, **put a picture on the door of your fridge that gives you inspiration** to stick to your plan. Underneath the picture, post the words, **"It's Your Choice,"** to remind you that you choose your reality and your level of success. It's really up to you.

# It's Your Choice!

**Today's Goodies:**

- Day 5 Meal Plan
- Avocado Salmon Tortilla Recipe
- Babaganush Recipe
- Daily Fitness & Diet Log

## EXERCISE DRILL—Day 5—Strengthen your Glutes

Today is rear-end day. (I am not kidding!)

**It is important to strengthen and maintain your glute muscles, as they tend to be more affected by gravity than any other part of our body**.

An easy way to strengthen your glutes without even having to leave your office chair is to contract your glutes (your bottom) 100 times in a row. Nobody will notice you are exercising and in no time, you will achieve great results.

As soon as you read this, contract your glutes 100 times in a row. You can decide to do a quick series and/or slow series, holding the "squeeze" longer each time as you see fit. DO THIS…It REALLY works!

You will see even greater results if you do this exercise several times a day.

Be strong!

## NUTRITIONAL TIP—Day 5- Start with Protein

Starting a meal with protein will help reduce the blood sugar surge that usually occurs after eating most refined carbohydrates (including snack bars, most breads, pasta, etc.). When your blood sugar increases, your body is more likely to store extra calories as fat at your next meal.

Physiologically, your body is constantly protecting your two major organs: your brain and your heart. Your brain needs fat (good fats) and your heart needs protein to function correctly. When your body receives carbohydrates first, a "message" about a potential lack of fat and protein is sent to your body's digestive system, and you will store more "fat" for use later. Why? Because your body feels most "comfortable" when it has a reserve of energy (glycogen).

Therefore, **the easiest way to prevent excess weight gain and to promote weight loss is to eat protein first,** followed by the remainder of your nutritionally balanced meal. This will ensure that the right message is sent to the brain and you will store less fat…

But beware: this is not a miracle trick. If you consume more calories than you expend (even if they do come from pure protein), you will still gain weight (and there are other medical ramifications of this approach, too), but not as much as if you had started your meal by eating pure, white sugar.

See you tomorrow,

*Valerie Your Private Coach*

# Meal Suggestions—Day 5

## 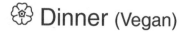 Breakfast (Vegan)

1 cup low-fat cottage cheese (or soy yogurt)
Stevia
1 cup strawberries
¼ honeydew melon

## Lunch

**\*Avocado Salmon Tortilla\***
1 orange

## Dinner (Vegan)

Middle Eastern plate: **\*Babaganush\***, **\*Hummus\***
1 whole-wheat pita bread
1 cup raspberries

# Avocado Salmon Tortilla

*. To satisfy your cravings for heavier, higher-fat foods, you can safely enjoy an Avocado Salmon Tortilla without any adverse diet effects.*
*. Avocado contains a proven property that lowers cholesterol.*
*. Salmon, like avocado, provides healthy fats (Omega-3), which also contribute to the lowering of LDL (bad) cholesterol.*

## Ingredients:

- 1 sprouted grains tortilla (the Ezekiel brand is a great buy)
- Half of a ripe avocado
- 1 teaspoon soyonnaise (to help keep the saturated fat at zero)
- Smoked wild salmon ~ to pu
- Lemon juice (optional)
- Salt to taste

## Directions:

-1- Warm tortilla in a hot skillet for 2 minutes.
-2- Put the tortilla on a plate.
-3- Spread soyonnaise and avocado on the tortilla and drizzle a few drops of lemon juice.
-4- Add a few thin pieces of salmon.
-5- Salt if needed.
-6- Fold ends and wrap it all up.

Enjoy!

Serves 1.

෴

# Babaganush

. Babaganush is a healthy dish that provides nearly all of your RDA of folacin (folic acid) and potassium. The typical American diet lacks these two critical nutrients.
. *Folacin is essential for the manufacture of genetic material as well as protein metabolism and red blood cell formation.*
. **Potassium helps maintain regular fluid balance. It's essential for nerve and muscle function.**

## Ingredients:

- 3 medium-sized eggplants
- 2 cloves of garlic
- ⅓ cup of olive oil
- Optional: 5 anchovy filets (from a can, in olive oil)
- Optional: mayonnaise or soyonnaise
- 1 lemon (juice)
- Salt to taste

## Directions:

-1- Poke holes in the eggplants using a fork.
-2- Cook them (one by one) in the microwave on high for 8 minutes.
-3- Cut them in half and scrape out the pulp (avoid the purple part as it does not taste good) into a food processor or blender.
-4- Add the lemon juice, anchovy filets, soyonnaise, garlic, olive oil and salt.
-5- Mix.

Serve cold with whole-wheat pita bread, hummus and a few olives, for a Middle Eastern combo plate.

Serves 4.

෨෪

# Daily Fitness & Diet Log

Date [                    ]

| | | | | |
|---|---|---|---|---|
| Overall Feeling Today: | ☺ ☺ ☹ | Overall Fitness: | ☺ ☺ ☹ |
| Overall Diet: | ☺ ☺ ☹ | Overall Stress Level: | ☺ ☺ ☹ |

## Diet...

| Breakfast | Lunch | Dinner |
|---|---|---|
| _____ | _____ | _____ |
| _____ | _____ | _____ |
| _____ | _____ | _____ |
| _____ | _____ | _____ |
| _____ | _____ | _____ |

Extra meal (if any): _____

Fluid Intake: [            ] cups. Type of fluid: _____

Trans fats?... yes / no     Refined carbs?... yes / no     Home-made food?... yes / no

## Fitness...

How many steps: [            ]

| | | | |
|---|---|---|---|
| Flexibility | ☑☒: _____ | ◷: _____ |
| MetaBoost | ☑☒: _____ | ◷: _____ |
| Strength | ☑☒: _____ | ◷: _____ |
| Cardio | ☑☒: _____ | ◷: _____ |
| Other | ☑☒: _____ | ◷: _____ |

# Day 6: Jump-Start (Days 3–7)

## Today is a beautiful day...Isn't life wonderful?

Keep reminding yourself throughout the day that you are dieting and exercising to improve your quality of life...you'll gain lots of energy! A healthy body! Increased stamina! It can't get much better than this.

**Today's Goodies:**

- Day 6 Meal Plan
- Daily Fitness & Diet Log

### EXERCISE DRILL—Day 6—Two at a Time

**Today, I encourage you to take the stairs whenever the opportunity arises...and when you do, take them two at a time.**

Concentrate on your form as you climb the stairs: stand tall, tighten your abs, and don't lean forward too much. **When you take the stairs two-by-two, you increase the load on your quadriceps (thighs) and on your glutes (butt),** which will add more definition and strength in the long run. By building muscle mass, you increase your metabolic rate, too.

If you are not in a situation where you feel comfortable taking the stairs two-by-two at this very moment, keep this tip in mind for when you are. It is THE secret to lean, strong thighs for a lifetime.

## NUTRITIONAL TIP—Day 6—Why Water?

Many toxins are released during the weight-loss process. The most effective way to flush these toxins out of your body is to drink lots and lots of water.

**You need an average of eight cups of water per day to make sure you eliminate the toxins you produce when you lose weight.** (See the intro for more information.) You can replace water with decaf tea and herbal teas. Water, however, cannot be replaced with sodas (too much sugar), diet sodas (artificial sweeteners can be harmful to your health), coffee or alcohol.

If you don't have a water bottle handy, go to your kitchen, nearest vending machine, or corner store and get one. And keep your water bottle in clear view throughout the day. **Drink at least one cup of room-temperature water (much better than freezing cold water) every 90 minutes.**

See you tomorrow,

*Valerie Your Private Coach*

# Meal Suggestions—Day 6

## ❀ Breakfast

2 slices whole-grain bread
4 slices smoked salmon 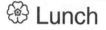 ~ Flavored tofu
1 apple

## ❀ Lunch

Garden salad with 3 tablespoons vinaigrette
Veggie burger patty
Whole-wheat bread
One apple

## ❀ Dinner (Vegan and Light)

1 bowl of light soup
1 plain yogurt (or soy yogurt)
Stevia

# Daily Fitness & Diet Log

Date

Overall Feeling Today: ☺ ☺ ☹          Overall Fitness:          ☺ ☺ ☹
Overall Diet: ☺ ☺ ☹          Overall Stress Level:          ☺ ☺ ☹

## Diet...

| Breakfast | Lunch | Dinner |
| --- | --- | --- |
| _____ | _____ | _____ |
| _____ | _____ | _____ |
| _____ | _____ | _____ |
| _____ | _____ | _____ |
| _____ | _____ | _____ |

Extra meal (if any): _____

Fluid Intake: [          ] cups. Type of fluid: _____

Trans fats?... yes / no          Refined carbs?... yes / no          Home-made food?... yes / no

## Fitness...                    How many steps: [          ]

Flexibility          ☑☒: _____          ⏰: _____

MetaBoost          ☑☒: _____          ⏰: _____

Strength          ☑☒: _____          ⏰: _____

Cardio          ☑☒: _____          ⏰: _____

Other          ☑☒: _____          ⏰: _____

# Day 7: Jump-Start (Days 3–7)

**Love yourself first...**

What do you feel towards yourself and your body? Do you choose to appreciate who you are, and what you contribute to others, or do you determine your self-worth by the number on the scale or what size jeans you wear?

**This might seem slightly ironic, but when you truly start loving yourself—from the inside, out—it seems as though the weight just naturally begins to melt away.**

Maybe it's because you love yourself enough to nourish your body with nutrient-rich foods, or because you love yourself enough not to pollute your body with toxins, additives and chemicals. Or maybe it's because you love yourself enough to give your body the physical exercise it needs to stay healthy and strong. Perhaps it's a combination of all three?

What can you do today to love yourself first? Give yourself permission to take care of your body! Remember, "it's your choice."

p.s. You have nearly completed your first week of BootCamp. Congratulations!

**Today's Goodies:**

- Day 7 Meal Plan
- Open-Face Tuna Sandwich Recipe
- TexMex Salad Recipe
- Miso Mushrooms Recipe
- Daily Fitness & Diet Log

This is the final day that you MUST follow all meal plans without making any changes or alterations (unless you have a specific medical condition). For the rest of the program, except days 15 and 16, you will have more flexibility. Isn't freedom of choice wonderful?

## EXERCISE DRILL—Day 7—Invisible Chair

You only need two minutes for this one…

Find a place with a flat wall where you can be by yourself. (If you work in an office, the restrooms work fine.)

To begin, lean your back flat against the wall, with your feet shoulder-width apart (approximately 15 inches) and approximately 12–16 inches from the wall. Slide down the wall until you look like you are sitting on an invisible chair. Your legs should be at a 90-degree angle (and you will feel your legs doing all of the work).

Make sure your back is flat and your knees don't go over your toes; otherwise, you may create unnecessary pressure in your knee joints.

Hold this position for ONE minute. If you don't have the strength to hold the position for an entire minute, repeat this exercise until you reach a total of ONE minute.

This is a great strength training exercise that helps, slowly but surely, build strong, sleek thighs.

Be strong!

## NUTRITIONAL TIP—Day 7—Eat real food instead of meal supplements

In the late 50s, the first meal replacement shakes were introduced by a company called "Metracal." Several competitors quickly jumped on the bandwagon as these meal replacement shakes gained popularity. However, very few people actually lost weight with these shakes, since a large number of dieters ate "normally" and finished their meal with a shake, thereby increasing their daily caloric intake!

A similar phenomenon continues to occur today. Although manufacturers claim that their products are well balanced and contain healthy fibers (which produce a "filling" effect), users tend to complain that they still feel hungry after drinking a diet shake…so much so that they tend to add "healthy-looking" snacks in between drinks. Regardless of whether they are healthy or not, these snacks add unwanted calories, and dieters fail to lose those extra pounds. This doesn't even take into account the fact that **most meal replacement shakes are filled with sugar**—something you want to avoid when dieting.

Besides, **I have yet to meet a single person who can keep up with the boredom and monotony of meals in a can.**

Snack bars are even more treacherous. Indeed, they are commonly advertised as "meal replacements." However, because they tend to be eaten quite quickly (usually in four bites), there is not enough time for the message of "fullness" to be sent to the brain. So, a second bar (or something more filling) is usually consumed right after the first bar. Furthermore, **a vast majority of these bars are loaded with saturated fat.** (Believe it or not, some bars endorsed by famous doctors provide a frightening 45% of your daily allowance for saturated fat in ONE BAR!) Plus, there are several ingredients with suspicious origins (genetically modified ingredients) and too many preservatives and artificial flavorings and colorings to count.

If you need to eat something in between meals, go for an apple or a slice of whole-wheat bread with low-fat cream cheese. All in all, go for something whose ingredients you can identify.

See you tomorrow,

*Valerie Your Private Coach*

# Meal Suggestions—Day 7

## 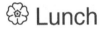 Breakfast (Light)

1 slice whole-grain bread
1 tablespoon strawberry preserve
5 strawberries

## 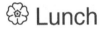 Lunch

**\*Open Face Tuna Sandwich\***
Salad mix + 3 tablespoons vinaigrette
1 apple

## 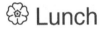 Dinner (Vegan)

**\*TexMex Salad\***
Gardenburger meatless riblets
\*Miso Mushrooms\*

# Open-Face Tuna Sandwich

**A quick recipe (five minutes to prepare at most), for those times where you are in a rush!**
**This healthy dish provides good omega fats, protein and fiber—enough to leave you full until the next meal.**

## Ingredients:

- 2 slices of whole-grain bread
- 1 small can of tuna in water ("no salt added" is best, to reduce the level of sodium in your diet)
- 2 tablespoons of soyonnaise (or real mayo if you cannot live without it)
- 3 tablespoons of balsamic vinegar
- Onion powder

## Directions:

-1- In a bowl, mix all ingredients: tuna, soyonnaise, vinegar and onion powder.
-2- Cut bread slices in half.
-3- Spread mixture on bread halves. You get 4 small, open-face sandwiches.
-4- Savor the taste of the food. Take your time when you eat.

## Variations:

If you have two more minutes, take the time to chop an onion and use fresh onion instead of onion powder.

და

# TexMex Salad

**. This is a great way to get your fiber for the day.**
**. Tuna provides omega-3 fats, which are proven to lower cholesterol.**

## Ingredients:

- 1 can pinto beans, drained and rinsed
- 1 can black beans, drained and rinsed
- 1 cup shredded cheddar cheese (or low-fat mozzarella for a lower count in saturated fat)
- 10 ounces of rinsed salad mix
- 1 large can of tuna
- Canola oil and red wine vinegar for the vinaigrette (or if in a hurry, use low-fat Catalina salad dressing)
- Salt and pepper, to taste
- Minced cilantro, to taste

## Directions:

**-1-** Mix all ingredients in a large salad bowl.
**-2-** Prepare vinaigrette and add sparingly to salad.

Serves 4.

Enjoy!

୫୦

# Miso Mushrooms Dish

. This original dish brings an Asian feel to your table.

. *Mushrooms provide a high level of* **selenium:** *an essential mineral that works closely with vitamin E to produce antioxidants that neutralize the cell-damaging "free radicals" that can increase the risk of cancer and other diseases caused by aging. It plays an important role in the immune system, the thyroid system and the male reproductive system.*

. *Mushrooms also provide* **potassium** *and* **copper, which** *is another essential mineral. Iron's role in making red blood cells and delivering oxygen to every part of the body is well-documented and understood. But did you know that iron couldn't do its job without copper?*

. **Mushrooms also contain three vitamins from the B group, including riboflavin, which promotes healthy skin and good vision.**

## Ingredients:

- 2 boxes of sliced mushrooms (crimini or white)
- Low-sodium soy sauce
- 1 packet of instant miso soup
- Canola oil
- No salt! (soy sauce and miso instant mix will bring plenty of it)

## Directions:

-1- Sauté mushrooms in canola oil over medium-high heat until ready to eat.
-2- Every 5 minutes during cooking, drizzle a few drops of soy sauce.
-3- When mushrooms are cooked, add 1/3 cup of water and the miso soup instant mix.
-4- Mix for 2 minutes or until water is almost all evaporated (keep enough for a nice sauce though).

That's it!

## Variations:

You can add tofu (which will provide additional calcium), or chicken for a lean source of animal protein, etc…

ꝏ

# Daily Fitness & Diet Log

Date [                    ]

Overall Feeling Today: ☺ ☺ ☹          Overall Fitness:        ☺ ☺ ☹
Overall Diet:          ☺ ☺ ☹          Overall Stress Level:   ☺ ☺ ☹

## Diet...

| Breakfast | Lunch | Dinner |
|---|---|---|
| _____ | _____ | _____ |
| _____ | _____ | _____ |
| _____ | _____ | _____ |
| _____ | _____ | _____ |
| _____ | _____ | _____ |

Extra meal (if any): _____

Fluid Intake: [            ] cups. Type of fluid: _____

Trans fats?... yes / no          Refined carbs?... yes / no          Home-made food?... yes / no

## Fitness...

How many steps: [            ]

Flexibility    ☑☒: _____    🕐: _____

MetaBoost      ☑☒: _____    🕐: _____

Strength       ☑☒: _____    🕐: _____

Cardio         ☑☒: _____    🕐: _____

Other          ☑☒: _____    🕐: _____

# Day 8: Energy Pump (Days 8–14)

**Welcome to Week 2 of BootCamp!**

It's time to **weigh yourself** this morning. If possible, use a scale that calculates body fat, which is a much better indicator of how fit or healthy you really are. Use the guidelines in the introduction to see how your body composition measures up.

It's time to get your energy pumping! **This week, you will be introduced to your first MetaBoost Card. Do the routine EVERY DAY (it only takes 5 minutes), in addition to your 30-minute walk on an empty stomach.** You can either do your MetaBoost Workout after your walk, or at any other time of the day. If you want to do it more than once, go for it! The more physical activity you do, the better. But at a minimum, do your MetaBoost Workout at least once per day.

To find out more about the MetaBoost Workouts, see the "Frequently Asked Questions" found at the end of this book.

**For the remainder of the program (except for days 15 and 16), you may choose what you want to eat for breakfast, lunch and dinner from the selection of meal plans you receive each week and the meal plans you previously received.**

Again, I strongly suggest that you do not alter the content of the meal plans themselves, but you can certainly mix and match your favorite meals day-by-day. Why? You will have a higher success rate on this program if you have freedom of choice. And by choosing your meals wisely, you will learn how to continue eating healthy, balanced meals well after this BootCamp is complete.

You will also find the "healthier" fast food choices with "Today's Goodies." These suggestions are only to be used when you truly have no time to prepare for the other meal plans.

By the way, if you do get hungry in between meals, you can have a small snack from the recommended "Healthy Snack List." But always have a glass of water first when you feel hungry and then wait at least 15 minutes to see if the hunger is still there. If it is, have a healthy snack. But eat no more than one snack per day.

Here we go!

**Today's Goodies:**

- Breakfast, Lunch and Dinner Meal Plans (Rotate with the meal plans from Week 1 for healthy variety and a bit of freedom, too.)
- Shopping List for Week 2
- Healthy Snack List
- "Healthier" Fast Food Choices List
- MetaBoost Workout #1
- Purple Milkshake Recipe
- Feta Olive Whole-Wheat Pasta Salad Recipe
- Three-Color Fruit Salad Recipe
- Daily Fitness & Diet Log

# EXERCISE DRILL—Day 8—Outer Thighs

Today we are going to work on your outer thighs (also known as your hip abductors).

Stand up and hold onto a shelf that is approximately chest height for balance. Stand on the leg that is closest to whatever you are holding on to.

Raise the leg that is extended out to the side to about 45 degrees, without moving or bouncing at the hips. Use a controlled movement, and lower the leg back down—without resting it on the floor. Remember to keep your abs tight.

Do 20 repetitions. Rest. Do 20 more. Now switch legs and do the same two sets on the other side (we have to keep those hips equal).

To make this more difficult, turn your toe inward slightly as you raise it out to the side. Feel the contraction in your outer thigh and glutes.

Do this at least two or three times per day today.

Be strong!

## NUTRITIONAL TIP—Day 8—Start An Apple Week

Here's a helpful tip that every healthy person should know…

We are going to start an apple week together this week. If you choose to continue this part of the program beyond the next seven days, great!

The concept is as simple as it gets: on your next trip to the grocery store or the farmers' market, purchase five pounds of organic apples. Starting today, begin each meal with an apple. Wait between 10 to 20 minutes before eating your "real" meal. You will be amazed at how much your appetite is reduced by the small apple.

What's the secret? Apples contain large amounts of pectin (a natural fiber), which naturally curbs your appetite. By eating one small apple before every meal, you will eat less at your next meal, and thus, throughout the day.

Go for it!

See you tomorrow,

*Valerie Your Private Coach*

# Meal Suggestions—Days 8 to 14

# Mix & Match

## ❀ Breakfast

| Choice #1—Vegetarian | Choice #2 | Choice #3 |
|---|---|---|
| 1 cup slow-cooked oatmeal<br>Stevia<br><br>2 tablespoons plain yogurt | 2 slices whole-grain bread<br>3 slices smoked salmon<br>1 cup blueberries | * Purple Milkshake *<br><br>1 egg + 1 strip of bacon<br><br>1 slice whole-grain bread |

## ❀ Lunch

| Choice #1—Vegan | Choice #2—Vegetarian | Choice #3—Vegetarian |
|---|---|---|
| 1 cup vegan chili<br><br>Spinach salad<br><br>1 cup strawberries | Spinach salad<br><br>* Feta Eggplant Caviar *<br><br>15 low-carb tortilla chips | * Feta Olive Whole-Wheat Pasta Salad *<br><br>* Three-Color Fruit Salad * |

## ❀ Dinner

| Choice #1 | Choice #2—Indian | Choice #3—Vegan |
|---|---|---|
| *Tomato Soup with Edamame*<br><br>*Olive Cumin Chicken*<br>1 apple | Chicken Tandoori and pea sauce<br><br>Raita<br><br>Cooked spinach | Combo: *hummus, babaganush, miso mushrooms*<br>1 slice whole-grain bread<br>1 small soy yogurt |

# ഇ **Shopping List—Week 2** ഇ

| **Vegetables, Legumes & Nuts** | **Fruit** |
|---|---|
| - Vegetarian chili<br>- 1 bunch spinach<br>- 8 large eggplants<br>- 2 medium-ripe tomatoes<br>- 2 onions<br>- Fresh parsley<br>- Pitted kalamata black olives<br>- Pitted green olives<br>- Basil leaves<br>- Mint leaves (optional)<br>- Tomato soup<br>- Edamame (cooked or not—if not, just boil for 5 minutes)<br>- Oregano<br>- Thyme & laurel<br>- 1 can of peeled tomatoes<br>- 1 can garbanzo beans<br>- 1 clove of garlic<br>- Sun-dried tomatoes | - 5 lbs organic apples for Apple Week<br>- 4 cups blueberries<br>- 4 cups strawberries<br>- 5 lemons<br>- 2 cups raspberries |

| **Eggs & Dairy** | **Meat, Fish & Tofu** |
|---|---|
| - 2 plain yogurt (or soy)<br>- 2 cups low-fat milk (or soy)<br>- 400 grams of feta cheese (low-fat, if possible) | - 1 small package of wild smoked salmon<br>- 1 organic chicken<br>- 1 soy yogurt<br>- anchovy filets (optional) |

| Oils & Sweets | Miscellaneous |
|---|---|
| - Olive oil<br>- Canola oil<br>- Canola oil spray | - Slow-cooked oatmeal<br>- Whole-grain bread (small loaf)<br>- Vanilla extract<br>- Low-carb tortilla chips<br>- Whole-grain tortellini<br>- Red wine vinegar<br>- Cumin<br>- Soyonnaise |

# ℘ **Snack List** ℘

A few facts on snacks:

**-1-** We don't have to snack. Though we are constantly bombarded by ads promoting snack bars, if we have a sedentary job, snacking is not a necessity.

**-2-** That being said, a snack should address two major needs: stop your hunger feeling and avoid cravings two hours later.

**-3-** Before snacking, drink a large glass of water to make sure your hunger is real and you are not mistaking it for thirst.

**-4-** Make sure your environment is packed with healthy, light snacks so that you are not tempted to go to the vending machine.

---

. A few strips of turkey jerky or 98% fat free beef jerky
. 1 cup of low-fat cottage cheese with Stevia
. 1 apple
. 1 serving of Soy yogurt
. 1 low-fat mozzarella stick with 10 almonds
. 1 slice of whole-grain bread with peanut butter
. 1 cup of cereals + 1 cup of skim milk
. 1 cup of blueberries and 10 walnuts
. Half a small pouch of peanut M&Ms (if there is nothing else and you are starving for real)
. Half a cantaloupe melon with a small slice of prosciutto
. 1 slice of whole-grain bread with low-fat cream cheese
. 1 cup of strawberries with 10 almonds
. Celery sticks with 1 tablespoon of soyonnaise
. 100 grams of low-fat kettle potato chips
. 1 glass of skim milk with 1 tablespoon of honey
. 1 peach
. 1 cup of blackberries
. 1 veggie patty with a slice of whole-grain bread
. 2 slices of honeydew melon
. Broccoli with 1 tablespoon of soyonnaise
. Cauliflower with 1 tablespoon of soyonnaise
. 10 olives and half a whole-wheat pita
. 1 cup of black tea with lemon
. 1 red pepper and hummus
. Homemade Chai tea: hot Chai (teabag) + skim milk + Stevia

# ಣ "Healthier" Fast Food Choices ಣ

Although I recommend avoiding fast-food restaurants as often as possible, I do understand that sometimes you might not have time to prepare a healthier meal, and may need to buy something on the run. Here is a list of "Healthier" Fast Food Choices for those days when you absolutely need it. Remember to always choose water (never sodas or fruit drinks) and NEVER "super-size" any of your meals at any fast-food restaurant.

**Subway:** Any 6-inch, "under 6 grams of fat" sub (no cheese, no fatty dressing, and no mayo).

**McDonald's:** 1 small hamburger with apple slices or with a small serving of French fries.

**Taco Bell or Del Taco:** Fresco Style Gordita Supreme® (Chicken) or the Fresco Style Fiesta Burrito (Chicken).

**All other hamburger chains (Burger King, Jack in the Box, Wendy's, In-N-Out, Carl's Jr.):** 1 plain "junior" hamburger with a small fries is okay occasionally.

**Baja Fresh:** I love it! Choose from their "Healthier Choice" selections. They have a sign indicating the nutritional content for several of their dishes.

**Una Mas:** Try the veggie burrito and guacamole.

**Quizno's:** The veggie sandwich is a good pick.

**Boston Market:** Go for a small piece (no more than 1/4 of a chicken) of their rotisserie chicken, leave the French fries and choose a large green salad with dressing on the side.

**Togo:** Choose any low-fat (no meatballs) sandwich. The avocado wrap is also very good.

**Pita Pit:** Try their Middle Eastern stuffed pita with hummus, babaganush and other veggie choices.

**Fast-food restaurants to avoid:**

**KFC:** Fried chicken is not healthy! (Unless you leave the fried skin on the side and only eat the meat.)

**Krispy Kreme:** Stay away! I know these doughnuts are yummy, but in this BootCamp, it is important to stay away from anything that is extremely sweet and loaded with fat...besides, who can eat only one Krispy Kreme?

**Dairy Queen:** If you must, go for the fat-free, no sugar products. Avoid the hamburgers.

**Dunkin' Donuts:** Stay away! (For the same reasons as Krispy Kreme).

**Arby's:** The vast majority of their dishes are loaded with fat and refined carbs. If you have no other option, go for a simple salad with dressing on the side, so that you can control how much fat you are ingesting.

# MetaBoost Workout #1 (5-Minute Drill)

For those of us who are pressed for time, there is always a way to squeeze in exercise, every single day.

It is important that you fit cardio, strength, flexibility, body alignment and de-stress training into your routine as often as possible.

This five-minute, metabolism-boosting workout has been created specifically for you. You can perform this routine several times throughout your day. The more often you move the better. This workout will help you boost your metabolism, which is what you need in order to lose weight for good!

## 5-Minute MetaBoost

1 min march in place (warm up)
1 min squats
1 min push ups
1 min abdominal crunches
1 min march in place (cool down)

Or

1 min march in place (warm up)
1 min jump rope
1 min lunges
1 min side to side leaps over a broom on the floor
1 min march in place (cool down)

Or

5-min power walk around the block

# Purple Milkshake

. This tasty, sweet, little pleasure is easy and quick to prepare.
. It provides a good amount of muscle-building proteins, and the blueberries make it rich in antioxidants.

## Ingredients:

2 cups fresh or slightly thawed blueberries
1 container (8 oz.) plain yogurt or soy yogurt
1 teaspoon powdered Stevia (or to taste)
5 drops of vanilla extract
2 cups milk or plain soy milk
1½ cups ice (or 16 cubes)

## Directions:

Put all the ingredients in the blender.
Vrrrrrrrrrrrrrrrrrrmmmmmmmmmmmmmmmmm…It's ready!

Serves 4.

## Variations:

You can replace the blueberries with strawberries, or apricots—in fact, you can use any berry or soft fruit you choose.

୫୬

# Feta Olive Whole-Wheat Pasta Salad

. **This interesting mix provides the vast majority of the nutrients we need from a meal: proteins, complex carbohydrates, dark, leafy greens, etc...**

. Whole-grain pasta provides much-needed vitamin B6, which is critical for the absorption of magnesium.

. Feta cheese provides protein and calcium (Did you know that 75% of adult Americans do not get their recommended daily amount [RDA] of calcium?)

## Ingredients:

- 2 cups whole-grain tortellini (cooked and refrigerated or room temperature)
- 10 pitted kalamata black olives, cut in half
- 10 (or to taste) basil leaves, rinsed, pat-dried and chopped
- 2 cups cubed feta cheese
- ½ cup olive oil
- 2 tablespoons red wine vinegar
- Salt and pepper to taste (keep in mind this dish already gets salt from the feta cheese, so make sure you taste it before adding any salt.)

## Directions:

-1- Mix all ingredients in a large salad bowl.
-2- Serve and enjoy right away.
-3- This is not a salad that can be kept for the following day, since pasta will absorb the dressing and become mushy.

Serves 6.

Enjoy!

## Variations:

As a blue cheese lover, I have tried this recipe with a little bit of blue cheese, and I loved it!

ℬℭ

# Three-Color Fruit Salad

*. In addition to folate, vitamin C, fiber and potassium, berries provide a high level of vitamin A, which helps maintain good vision, especially night vision.*
**. This quickly prepared salad will provide powerful phytochemicals—like flavonoids that have anti-inflammatory properties—which will make your skin look great.**
*. In addition, berries are charged with antioxidants, which provide protection by neutralizing free radicals—substances in the body that can damage cells and lead to disease.*

## Ingredients:

- 1 pint of strawberries (fresh)
- 1 pint of raspberries (fresh or frozen)
- ½ pint of blueberries (fresh or frozen)
- 1 squeezed lemon
- Stevia
- Mint leaves (for decoration and taste)

## Directions:

**-1-** Rinse all berries.
**-2-** Defrost the frozen berries in your microwave or, even better, take them out of the freezer two hours before using them.
**-3-** Cut the strawberries in half or in quarters, depending on size.
**-4-** Put them in a salad bowl.
**-5-** Add the blueberries and mix.
**-6-** Mix ½ of the raspberries in a mixer and blend.
**-7-** Add blended raspberries and whole raspberries to the fruit salad.
**-8-** Add lemon juice.
**-9-** Stir gently with a spoon.
**-10-** Add Stevia to taste.
**-11-** Decorate with mint leaves.

Enjoy!

Serves 4.

## Variations:

You can top with plain yogurt whipped with Stevia.

❧

# Daily Fitness & Diet Log

Date [ ]

| | | | |
|---|---|---|---|
| Overall Feeling Today: | ☺ ☹ ☺ | Overall Fitness: | ☺ ☹ ☺ |
| Overall Diet: | ☺ ☹ ☺ | Overall Stress Level: | ☺ ☹ ☺ |

## Diet...

| Breakfast | Lunch | Dinner |
|---|---|---|
| _____ | _____ | _____ |
| _____ | _____ | _____ |
| _____ | _____ | _____ |
| _____ | _____ | _____ |
| _____ | _____ | _____ |

Extra meal (if any): _____

Fluid Intake: [ ] cups. Type of fluid: _____

Trans fats?... yes / no          Refined carbs?... yes / no          Home-made food?... yes / no

## Fitness...                    How many steps: [ ]

| | | |
|---|---|---|
| Flexibility | ☑☒: _____ | ○: _____ |
| MetaBoost | ☑☒: _____ | ○: _____ |
| Strength | ☑☒: _____ | ○: _____ |
| Cardio | ☑☒: _____ | ○: _____ |
| Other | ☑☒: _____ | ○: _____ |

# Day 9: Energy Pump (Days 8–14)

## How are you today?

What did you think of your first MetaBoost workout? It's EASY and FAST and yet so EFFECTIVE!

You're doing great…I am rooting for you!

## EXERCISE DRILL—Day 9—Defined Calves

Here's a tip to help add definition to your calves…

Before climbing a flight of stairs, stand on the first step, with your heels hanging over the edge. Point your toes so that you're standing on your tiptoes; hold, and release, allowing your heels to come down a little bit lower than the height of the stair.

Do a quick set of 20 calf-raises before climbing the flight of stairs, and do another quick set at the top.

If you do this every time you climb a flight of stairs, you will start seeing results in no time. (Remember to choose the stairs over the elevator whenever possible, too.)

Be strong!

## NUTRITIONAL TIP—Day 9—Eat Your Greens

When compared to regular-leaf lettuce, romaine lettuce and butterhead lettuce, spinach comes out on top for nutritional content.

**Spinach has three times more calcium, three times more iron, eight times more magnesium, and more than two times more phosphorus and zinc, than other types of lettuce.**

What does this mean for you? You don't have to eat nearly the same amount of spinach to get the same nutritional benefits from these other vegetables…and since we can't eat salad all day, every day, we might as well get as many nutrients as we can at one sitting.

Enjoy!

*Valerie Your Private Coach*

# Daily Fitness & Diet Log

Date

Overall Feeling Today:    ☺ ☺ ☹          Overall Fitness:          ☺ ☺ ☹
Overall Diet:             ☺ ☺ ☹          Overall Stress Level:     ☺ ☺ ☹

## Diet...

| Breakfast | Lunch | Dinner |
|-----------|-------|--------|
|           |       |        |

Extra meal (if any): _____

Fluid Intake: [        ] cups. Type of fluid: _____

Trans fats?... yes / no        Refined carbs?... yes / no        Home-made food?... yes / no

## Fitness...                    How many steps: [        ]

Flexibility      ☑☒: _____    🕐: _____

MetaBoost        ☑☒: _____    🕐: _____

Strength         ☑☒: _____    🕐: _____

Cardio           ☑☒: _____    🕐: _____

Other            ☑☒: _____    🕐: _____

# Day 10: Energy Pump (Days 8–14)

## We're a third of the way there!

Having a positive attitude will greatly affect your success rate. If your thoughts are going something like this: "Oh no, twenty days to go!" STOP! And look at the progress you're making instead of the gap between where you are and where you want to be. When you focus on your accomplishments, you will build on your success and keep going.

There is always a bright side of life. Success breeds success and the momentum continues to accelerate.

### EXERCISE DRILL—Day 10—Get that Heart Pumping

Do you spend long hours at your desk? Here's an easy tip to keep you energized throughout your day.

**Set an alarm at your desk to beep every 60 minutes. When you hear the "beep," get up and jog for 90 seconds on the spot.** If you're wearing high heels, take them off. If you're embarrassed to do this in your office, go to the restroom to do it. If you're in a two-hour meeting and cannot be interrupted, go to the restrooms after the meeting and jog in place for three full minutes to make up for the minute and a half you lost.

You will keep your blood pumping and your cardiovascular system will improve, too. This will increase your alertness and motivation and will decrease the "sluggish" feeling that is so common in the afternoon…not to mention that **you will have added at least an extra 15 minutes of exercise to your day.**

Be strong!

## NUTRITIONAL TIP—Day 10—Look out sweeteners, here comes Stevia!

Beware of sweeteners; not all sweeteners are created alike.

Sweeteners are continuously being developed, as more and more people continue to diet. It is now possible to find NutraSweet™ in the most remote region of Mongolia! (But remember, some sweeteners—like aspartame, for example—may have harmful side effects from a health perspective.)

So how do you tame your sweet tooth? Should you use regular sugar and honey instead of sweeteners? I have been studying what's on the market for the past year and I have come to the following conclusion:

**The only no-calorie, all-natural sweetener that does not impact your blood sugar and which has no bitter taste is called Stevia.** In many places throughout the world, Stevia can be found in the sweeteners section of local grocery stores. However, in the USA, because of very efficient lobbying from mainstream sweeteners manufacturers, Stevia can only be found in the supplements section of select stores.

Our suggestion is to replace sweeteners in your diet with Stevia, as I do not believe that humans should consume anything artificial in their diets. According to several serious medical studies Stevia offers a safe, all-natural alternative to other "toxic time-bombs."

See you tomorrow,

*Valerie Your Private Coach*

# Daily Fitness & Diet Log

Date [        ]

Overall Feeling Today:  ☺ ☺ ☹      Overall Fitness:        ☺ ☺ ☹
Overall Diet:           ☺ ☺ ☹      Overall Stress Level:   ☺ ☺ ☹

## Diet...

Breakfast                Lunch                    Dinner

_____        _____         _____

_____        _____         _____

_____        _____         _____

_____        _____         _____

_____        _____         _____

Extra meal (if any): _____

Fluid Intake: [        ] cups. Type of fluid: _____

Trans fats?... yes / no      Refined carbs?... yes / no      Home-made food?... yes / no

## Fitness...                          How many steps: [        ]

Flexibility    ☑☒: _____    ◷: _____

MetaBoost      ☑☒: _____    ◷: _____

Strength       ☑☒: _____    ◷: _____

Cardio         ☑☒: _____    ◷: _____

Other          ☑☒: _____    ◷: _____

# Day 11: Energy Pump (Days 8–14)

**It's a beautiful life...**And the weight just keeps dropping!

By following my guidelines, your energy should improve while the pounds keep on dropping. Consider this a friendly reminder to go for your 30-minute walk, do your MetaBoost workout, drink at least eight glasses of water, and move for at least 60 minutes throughout your day. These are simple, basic tips that really work.
Keep up the great work! Go, go, go!

## EXERCISE DRILL—Day 11—Improve your Posture

It's time to work on your posture. Sit straight, stand tall, SMILE.

**Your posture is a critical factor in your health and well-being. Better posture not only decreases back pain, but it also increases confidence.** How? As we stand tall and strong, we naturally project confidence—especially as we age. Those who develop good posture at an early age rarely experience aches and pains in their backs later in life. Having the ability to maintain an active lifestyle as we age certainly does improve confidence as well.

For this exercise, find a wall and stand with your back and your heels right against the wall. If you are wearing high-heeled shoes, please remove them before doing this exercise.

Pull your shoulders back so that they are against the wall, too. Now your heels, your bottom, your back and your shoulders should all be against the wall.

Raise your arms in front of you slowly, until they are as high up as you can reach them without arching your back. Try to touch your thumbs to the wall above your head. If you can do that, you have superb posture. If you have a hard time reaching the wall above without arching your back, then keep practicing. By performing this exercise daily, you will gradually improve your posture, and decrease the risk of back pain and/or degenerative back problems.

Breathe out as you raise your arms. Breathe in as you lower them. Do this exercise 15 times. Rest and repeat the entire set.

Repeat the sequence at least three times throughout the day.

Be strong!

## NUTRITIONAL TIP—Day 11—Choose Strawberry

Here's a simple, yet interesting tip…

Of all the types of jams or other fruit preserves out there, when consumed, **strawberry jam raises your blood sugar level the least.** This isn't an invitation to eat strawberry jam by the spoonful, but if you are going to put a fruit preserve on your toast, *choose strawberry!*

A teaspoonful of strawberry jam is also a delicious treat in a serving of plain, non-fat yogurt.

See you tomorrow,

*Valerie Your Private Coach*

# Daily Fitness & Diet Log

Date [ ]

Overall Feeling Today: ☺ 😐 ☹  Overall Fitness: ☺ 😐 ☹
Overall Diet: ☺ 😐 ☹  Overall Stress Level: ☺ 😐 ☹

## Diet...

| Breakfast | Lunch | Dinner |
|---|---|---|
| ______ | ______ | ______ |
| ______ | ______ | ______ |
| ______ | ______ | ______ |
| ______ | ______ | ______ |
| ______ | ______ | ______ |

Extra meal (if any): ______

Fluid Intake: [ ] cups. Type of fluid: ______

Trans fats?... yes / no  Refined carbs?... yes / no  Home-made food?... yes / no

## Fitness...

How many steps: [ ]

| | | |
|---|---|---|
| Flexibility | ☑☒: ______ | 🕓: ______ |
| MetaBoost | ☑☒: ______ | 🕓: ______ |
| Strength | ☑☒: ______ | 🕓: ______ |
| Cardio | ☑☒: ______ | 🕓: ______ |
| Other | ☑☒: ______ | 🕓: ______ |

# Day 12: Energy Pump (Days 8–14)

## Creatures of Habit...

You may have noticed that you are a creature of habit. Most of us are! Many of the things you do each day are a part of a pattern you have developed that you consider "normal."

You probably set your alarm at the same time each morning; get up out of the same side of the bed; use the same toothpaste; put your tooth-brush in the same spot; wash your hair and body the same way; sit at the same seat at the table; take the same route to your office or to the gym or to the grocery store—wherever you go on a regular basis. You may even switch lanes at the same places en route to where you want to go. You'll answer the phone in the same way; sign your messages with the same greeting; go to the same places with your friends; and probably order the same thing on the menu. You get the picture, right? In a nutshell, **a habit is something you do over and over again, and don't question, because that's just the way things are. Habits are the things we just "do."**

What you may not recognize is the profound impact that your habits have on your results. **The ability to become aware of your current habits and to create new habits to support your vision will be paramount to your success.**

By the way, **creating new habits and awareness is the foundation of this program. Without even knowing it, you are developing the** *habit* **of walking in the morning, the** *habit* **of preparing your meals, and the** *habit* **of doing a MetaBoost workout every day.**

It takes approximately 28 days for a new habit to develop. After 30 days on this program, you should have developed most of these successful weight-loss habits. And it will be up to you to choose what to do with them…

## EXERCISE DRILL—Day 12—Flat Abs

**Think about holding in your lower and upper abs at all times when you walk today.** You might consider wearing something around your wrist (like a special bracelet or a favorite watch), as a structure to remind to hold in your abs throughout the day.

This will help work the deep abdominal muscles that no crunches can reach!

This will also help you create a flat stomach without any sweating required :o)

Remember to hold in your stomach and to contract your abdominal muscles as often as you can.

Be strong!

## NUTRITIONAL TIP—Day 12—Going Back to Our Roots

From 1900 to 1976, fat consumption in the Western world rose by 25%, with most coming from saturated fat. Sadly, that number keeps rising.

Ask yourself…

- **Do you opt for potato chips over wild roots?**
- **Do you prefer wild rice or puffed rice?**
- **Do you eat apricot jam or fresh apricots?**
- **How often do you quench your thirst with mountain spring water instead of sweetened, caffeinated, or chemical brews?**

- **If you have to decide between French fries and spinach, hot dogs and legumes, or fruit-flavored candy and grapes, what do you choose?**
- **Do you know the difference between a wild grain and a processed grain?**
- **Do you eat wild meat?**
- **When was the last time you ate veggies as a main course, instead of just a side dish?**

You can see that our choices for foods have changed enormously over the past 100 years. **Choose a more natural, plant-based diet more often, and you will greatly improve your health, and naturally slim down your waistline.**

Make it a great day,

*Valerie Your Private Coach*

# Daily Fitness & Diet Log

Date [                    ]

Overall Feeling Today:   ☺ ☺ ☹          Overall Fitness:        ☺ ☺ ☹
Overall Diet:            ☺ ☺ ☹          Overall Stress Level:   ☺ ☺ ☹

## Diet...

| Breakfast | Lunch | Dinner |
| --- | --- | --- |
| _____ | _____ | _____ |
| _____ | _____ | _____ |
| _____ | _____ | _____ |
| _____ | _____ | _____ |
| _____ | _____ | _____ |

Extra meal (if any): _____

Fluid Intake: [          ] cups. Type of fluid: _____

Trans fats?... yes / no        Refined carbs?... yes / no        Home-made food?... yes / no

## Fitness...                How many steps: [          ]

Flexibility    ☑☒: _____    ◷: _____

MetaBoost      ☑☒: _____    ◷: _____

Strength       ☑☒: _____    ◷: _____

Cardio         ☑☒: _____    ◷: _____

Other          ☑☒: _____    ◷: _____

# Day 13: Energy Pump (Days 8–14)

**Good morning!**

Have you ever noticed that how you do anything is how you do every-thing?

Some people have a hard time completing a task; other people refuse to take risks; others slow right down before the finish line even though they always complete the task; and then there are those who focus on only one thing at a time; and still others who can't seem to focus on ANYTHING for any length of time.

Have you noticed this about people? And have you also noticed that most people don't have one personality one day, and then switch to another one the next? They are either tried-and-true procrastinators, or true-blooded risk takers, but rarely both.

Sure, you might say for yourself that, "it depends on the situation," but **if you really pay close attention to the way you do things, you'll notice that how you do anything is how you do everything.**

But you can change the way you do things and train yourself to a new way of life. You can choose the life you want to live.

So how do you want to "be" on this program? Successful? Energetic? Committed to the end?

Keep up the great work...I am here with you all the way!

## EXERCISE DRILL—Day 13—Strong Arms

Another day for your triceps.

After your 5-minute MetaBoost drill today, find two weights (you can use canned food or milk jugs if you don't have weights) and **get ready to work your triceps again.** (Do this strength-building exercise after your MetaBoost drill because the muscles will have been warmed up by the previous exercise.)

Hold on to your weights in both hands and stand with your feet shoulder-width apart, abs tight. Bend forward slightly at the waist. Pull your arms back so that the upper parts of your arms are in alignment with your torso, and your elbows are bent.
Push the weights back to straighten your arms and feel the contraction in your triceps. Return to the starting position. Repeat the movement 20 times and then rest.

Do three sets of 20.

Remember, if you really want to continue working your triceps, do your standing push-ups every time you go to the restrooms today, too. Be strong!

## NUTRITIONAL TIP—Day 13
## Oatmeal...Does it Matter What Kind?

When choosing between slow-cooked or instant oatmeal, always choose slow-cooked.

Why? **Slow-cooked oatmeal has a much lower glycemic index than instant oatmeal. Therefore, it has a lower impact on your blood sugar.** When your blood sugar goes up too high, too fast, your body stores more energy as fat on the subsequent meal. Instant oatmeal has been precooked and the process of precooking makes it a fast carb.

Interesting how just the type of oatmeal you choose can have such an impact on your waistline.

See you tomorrow,

*Valerie Your Private Coach*

# Daily Fitness & Diet Log

Date [          ]

Overall Feeling Today: ☺ ☺ ☹          Overall Fitness: ☺ ☺ ☹
Overall Diet: ☺ ☺ ☹                    Overall Stress Level: ☺ ☺ ☹

## Diet...

| Breakfast | Lunch | Dinner |
|---|---|---|
| _____ | _____ | _____ |
| _____ | _____ | _____ |
| _____ | _____ | _____ |
| _____ | _____ | _____ |
| _____ | _____ | _____ |

Extra meal (if any): _____

Fluid Intake: [          ] cups. Type of fluid: _____

Trans fats?... yes / no          Refined carbs?... yes / no          Home-made food?... yes / no

## Fitness...                    How many steps: [          ]

Flexibility          ☑☒: _____          ◷: _____

MetaBoost            ☑☒: _____          ◷: _____

Strength             ☑☒: _____          ◷: _____

Cardio               ☑☒: _____          ◷: _____

Other                ☑☒: _____          ◷: _____

# Day 14: Energy Pump (Days 8–14)

## Eat Organic Whenever Possible!

Did you know that **the average North American consumes any-where from 135 to 150 pounds of sugar, food additives, chemicals and preservatives per year?**

That's an enormous amount of nutritional "junk" that we're putting into our bodies!
At their best, additives and artificial ingredients simply add little or no nutritional value to a food product. At their worst, additives pose a threat to your health. Side effects include lethargy, exhaustion, headaches, interrupted sleep, and in worst-case scenarios, cancer and other terminal diseases.

**Just because the FDA does not consider an additive "harmful" does not mean that it is safe to eat or that it has no side effects. At the same time, just because a certain food product is sold at the supermarket or is included in prepackaged foods or restaurant fare does not mean it is nutritionally good for you either.**

Does that mean you can avoid these substances all together? No. That would be nearly impossible. But you can make educated choices when you shop. Buy organic whenever possible and read your food labels to avoid extra additives and preservatives in your food.

And one more thing: **avoid refined sugar whenever possible. It is one of the most widely used food additives out there.**

## EXERCISE DRILL—Day 14- Streeeeeetch

Today we will focus on FLEXIBILITY.

What is flexibility, and why is it important?

**Flexibility increases physical efficiency and performance.** When you have flexible muscles, you are able to move through a particular range of motion with much more ease and efficiency.

Not only that, **flexibility decreases risk of injury, increases blood supply and nutrients to your joints, provides increased quality and quantity of joint synovial fluid (the lubricant within the joints), increases neuromuscular coordination and balance, and reduces muscle soreness after exercise.**

Sounds good, doesn't it?

Here's your assignment for today:

**-1-** Stand up and place one leg in front of the other with your forward heel down on the floor. Bend your knees and push your bottom back to feel the stretch in the **hamstrings** (back of the leg) of your forward leg. Hold for 30 seconds. Switch legs. Repeat.

**-2-** Now find a doorway. Grip the doorway with one hand, thumb facing up. Turn away from the doorway. Feel the stretch in your **chest and bicep** muscles. Hold for 30 seconds. Switch arms. Repeat.

**-3-** Next, stand up straight, feet shoulder-width apart. Lift one arm over your head and bend at the waist to the opposite side. Feel the stretch in your **waist**. Hold for 30 seconds. Switch sides. Repeat.

**-4-** And finally, find a friend to stretch with, and sit facing one another on the floor with the bottoms of your feet touching together. Hold hands and take turns pulling one another forward to get a nice, easy stretch through your **lower back**. When it's your turn for the stretch, close your eyes and breathe out, lowering your body as close to the floor as possible. Hold each stretch for 30 seconds.

Great work! You have taken steps to increase your flexibility today!

Keep it up every day and be strong!

## NUTRITIONAL TIP—Day 14—Go for Whole Grains

When it comes to breads and cereals, whole grains are the way to go. It takes longer for your body to digest whole grains; therefore, they have a lower impact on your blood sugar level, and you store less energy as fat at your next meal.

Furthermore, chewing signals a feeling of fullness to the brain (another reason why meal replacement shakes don't work), so you eat less and feel more satisfied.

If you love bread, European whole-grain bread is the better choice for a low glycemic index and pure satisfaction.

See you tomorrow,

*Valerie Your Private Coach*

# Daily Fitness & Diet Log

Date [        ]

Overall Feeling Today: ☺ ☺ ☹          Overall Fitness: ☺ ☺ ☹
Overall Diet: ☺ ☺ ☹                   Overall Stress Level: ☺ ☺ ☹

## Diet...

| Breakfast | Lunch | Dinner |
|-----------|-------|--------|
| _____ | _____ | _____ |
| _____ | _____ | _____ |
| _____ | _____ | _____ |
| _____ | _____ | _____ |
| _____ | _____ | _____ |

Extra meal (if any): _____

Fluid Intake: [        ] cups. Type of fluid: _____

Trans fats?... yes / no          Refined carbs?... yes / no          Home-made food?... yes / no

## Fitness...                    How many steps: [        ]

Flexibility   ☑☒: _____   🕐: _____

MetaBoost    ☑☒: _____   🕐: _____

Strength     ☑☒: _____   🕐: _____

Cardio       ☑☒: _____   🕐: _____

Other        ☑☒: _____   🕐: _____

# Day 15: Prep Day

**Welcome to Week 3 of BootCamp! You've reached the halfway point. Congratulations on your commitment to yourself and to this program.**

Please **weigh yourself** and log your results in your **"Ultimate Daily Fitness and Diet Log."**

We're going to start Week 3 with another cleanse—the RED CLEANSE™. We will prepare the body for tomorrow's cleanse with a light day today. Please note that you will need your juicer again for Day 16. Our favorite is the Breville Juice Fountain. (You can buy yours online at: http://www.myprivatecoach.com/store.)

## Follow the meal plans for Day 15 and 16 without alteration.

**You will also get your second MetaBoost Card this week. Do the routine EVERY DAY (MetaBoost Workout #2 only takes 10 minutes.) on top of your 30-minute walk on an empty stomach.** You can either do your MetaBoost Workout after your walk, or at any other time of the day. If you want to do it more than once, go for it. The more physical activity you do, the better. But at a minimum, do your MetaBoost Workout at least once per day.

**Today's Goodies:**

- Day 15 Meal Plan
- Day 16 RED CLEANSE™ Plan
- Breakfast, Lunch and Dinner Meal Plans for Days 17–21 (Rotate with the meal plans from Weeks 1 and 2 for healthy variety. Now you have a lot of choices!)

- Shopping List for Week 3
- MetaBoost Workout #2
- Artichoke with Yogurt Sauce Recipe
- Sweet Red Boost Recipe
- Savory Red Boost Recipe
- Sweet Dreams Red Boost Recipe
- Tomato, Arugula and Avocado Sandwich Recipe
- Mushroom Arugula Salad with Raisins Recipe
- Daily Fitness & Diet Log

## EXERCISE DRILL—Day 15—Taking care of Gravity

It's "Glutes Day" again today.

To continue our quest against gravity, **do your regular 100 "glute con-tractions," but this time focus on one side at a time.** This will isolate the muscles even more, and will ensure that each side gets the attention it deserves.

Nobody will notice you are exercising and in no time, you will achieve great results. Do this NOW! Keep your back straight and strong while you do your exercises. You can even do this while you read your e-mails.

Repeat this exercise several times a day. Remember, more is better.

## NUTRITIONAL TIP—Day 15—Farmers' Markets

**A farmers' market is a vending site in which farmers, growers or producers from a defined local area are present in person to sell their own produce and products, direct to the public. All products sold should have been grown, reared, caught, brewed, pickled, baked, smoked or processed by the stallholder.**

You will find that the vast majority of the produce at these markets is organic. In addition, you can also find several pre-packaged raw, vegan and vegetarian dishes. Going to a farmers' market obviously supports your local community, but it also creates the simple joy of being able to touch what you buy (as opposed to buying plastic boxes full of genetically modified, all perfect-looking veggies).

**Purchasing your produce at the markets will also help you stay in tune with the seasons.** As a Weight-Loss Coach, I believe that eating what Mother Nature has intended for us at certain times during the year makes more sense.

**Buying produce that was hand-picked the very morning of your purchase will also guarantee a high level of potent nutrients.** This is not true with the veggies and fruits that sit in supermarkets for days, or even weeks. (Sometimes longer!) Finally, you will interact with more people when you go to a farmers' market. Much more than when you go to your local supermarket, which makes the social aspect of the markets fun, too.

Enjoy the outdoors, enjoy touching what you buy, enjoy testing and tasting, enjoy life, and enjoy meeting new people...Isn't life beautiful?

See you tomorrow,

*Valerie Your Private Coach*

# Meal Suggestions—Day 15—Light

## 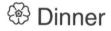 Breakfast

2 slices whole-grain bread
1 avocado
1 cup strawberries

## ❀ Lunch

**\*Arugula, Mushroom and Raisin Salad\***

## ❀ Dinner

1 bowl light soup
1 plain yogurt
Stevia

# Meal Suggestions—Day 16
# Red Cleanse™

## ✿ Breakfast

1 8-oz. glass **\*Sweet Red Boost\***

## ✿ Mid-Morning

Fresh mint tea

## ✿ Lunch

1 8-oz. glass **\*Savory Red Boost\***

## ✿ Mid-Afternoon

1 cup of Decaf Black Tea

## ✿ Dinner

1 8-oz. glass **\*Sweet Dreams Red Boost\***

## ✿ Before Bedtime

1 cup of Chamomile Tea

# Meal Suggestions—Days 17 to 21

# Mix & Match

## ❀ Breakfast

| Choice #1 | Choice #2 | Choice #3 |
|---|---|---|
| 2 slices whole-grain bread<br>Salmon-flavored cream cheese<br>1 cup strawberries | 2 slices whole-grain bread<br><br>2 slices smoked salmon<br><br>¼ honeydew | 1 cup GoLean Crunch cereal<br>1 cup soy milk<br>1 cup raspberries |

## ❀ Lunch

| Choice #1 | Choice #2 | Choice #3—Light |
|---|---|---|
| **\*Tomato Arugula and Avocado Sandwich\***<br><br>1 yogurt | 2 slices smoked salmon + whole-grain toast<br>Salad mix + 3 tablespoons vinaigrette<br>1 pear | **\*Hummus\***<br>15 low-carb chips<br>**\*Mushroom, Arugula, Chickpeas Salad\*** |

## ❀ Dinner

| Choice #1 | Choice #2 | Choice #3 - Vegetarian |
|---|---|---|
| Grilled chicken<br>**\*Provencale Ratatouille\***<br>1 cup low-fat Greek yogurt | Grilled antelope steak<br>Arugula salad with 3 tablespoons vinaigrette<br>1 apple | **\*Bean salad\***<br>**Grilled Chicken**<br>**1 Pear** |

# ဢ **Shopping List—Week 3** ဢ

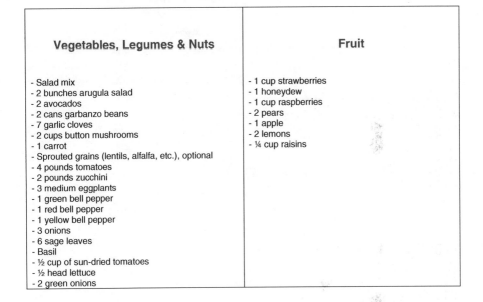

### Vegetables, Legumes & Nuts

- Salad mix
- 2 bunches arugula salad
- 2 avocados
- 2 cans garbanzo beans
- 7 garlic cloves
- 2 cups button mushrooms
- 1 carrot
- Sprouted grains (lentils, alfalfa, etc.), optional
- 4 pounds tomatoes
- 2 pounds zucchini
- 3 medium eggplants
- 1 green bell pepper
- 1 red bell pepper
- 1 yellow bell pepper
- 3 onions
- 6 sage leaves
- Basil
- ½ cup of sun-dried tomatoes
- ½ head lettuce
- 2 green onions

### Fruit

- 1 cup strawberries
- 1 honeydew
- 1 cup raspberries
- 2 pears
- 1 apple
- 2 lemons
- ¼ cup raisins

### Eggs & Dairy

- Salmon-flavored cream cheese
- 1 yogurt
- 1 low-fat Greek yogurt
- Grated parmesan cheese (optional)
- 1 egg
- ¼ cup blue cheese

### Meat, Fish & Tofu

- 1 small package of wild salmon
- Soy milk
- Grilled chicken (preferably organic)
- 1 antelope steak
- 200 grams of firm tofu (preferably organic)
- 2 slices bacon or tofu equivalent (the tofu equivalent is cholesterol-free and very tasty)
- 1 cup chopped, cooked chicken meat

| Oils & Sweets | Miscellaneous |
|---|---|
| - Olive oil<br>- Canola oil<br>- Canola oil spray | - Whole-grain bread (small loaf)<br>- 1 box GoLean Crunch! cereal<br>- Low-carb chips<br>- Dijon mustard<br>- Soyonnaise or mayonnaise<br>- Tahini paste (sesame)<br>- Cumin<br>- 1 cup of wild rice<br>- Broth: veggie or chicken<br>- Reduced-sodium soy sauce |

# MetaBoost Workout #2 (10-Minute Drill)

For those of us who are pressed for time, there is always a way to squeeze in exercise, every single day.

It is important that you fit cardio, strength, flexibility, body alignment and de-stress training into your routine as often as possible.

This 10-minute, metabolism-boosting workout has been created specifically for you. You can perform this routine several times throughout your day. The more often you move the better. This workout will help you boost your metabolism, which is what you need in order to lose weight for good.

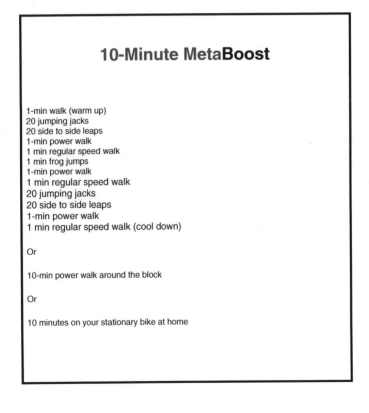

## 10-Minute Meta**Boost**

1-min walk (warm up)
20 jumping jacks
20 side to side leaps
1-min power walk
1 min regular speed walk
1 min frog jumps
1-min power walk
1 min regular speed walk
20 jumping jacks
20 side to side leaps
1-min power walk
1 min regular speed walk (cool down)

Or

10-min power walk around the block

Or

10 minutes on your stationary bike at home

# Yogurt Sauce for Artichoke

. This sauce is a delicious dip to accompany your artichoke without the fat of a regular oil/vinegar sauce.
. It is a healthy source of protein, too.

## Ingredients:

- 1 cup of plain fat-free yogurt or plain soy yogurt
- 2 teaspoons balsamic vinegar
- A dash of mustard or horseradish sauce
- Pepper and salt to taste
- Oregano (optional)

## Directions:

-1- Whip the yogurt with a plastic whip.
-2- Add mustard/horseradish.
-3- Add pepper and salt (and oregano, if you wish).
-4- Mix.
-5- Add the vinegar.
-6- Mix.

And voila!

## Variations:

You can add bits of blue cheese to bring a nice new taste to your artichoke.

℘

# Sweet Red Boost

. For this drink, you will need your juicer.
. **The Sweet Red Boost provides several much-needed nutrients and phyto-chemicals. Indeed:**
. **You will get your daily vitamin C recommended by the FDA, thanks to the apple, orange, strawberries and raspberries in this drink.**
. Strawberries provide a high level of manganese and vitamin K, along with potent phenols (antioxidants), which make it an "anti-cancer" fruit.
. Raspberries also provide a high level of manganese (necessary for proper brain function) and fiber that will help the digestive process.

## Ingredients:

- 1 apple
- 1 orange
- 1 cup strawberries
- 4 cups raspberries

## Directions:

-1- Rinse and pat dry all fruits/veggies. You can put your fruits directly in the juicer—no need to peel.
-2- Juice and drink right away, as antioxidants lose their potency as time passes.

Enjoy!

&

# Savory Red Boost

. For this drink, you will need your juicer.

. **The Savory Red Boost provides several much-needed nutrients and phyto-chemicals:**

- Celery is a good source of vitamin C, which helps support the immune system.

- **Carrots are the champions when it comes to vitamin A (1 cup = 800% of your recommended daily intake) and vitamin K (200% of your RDA). Additionally, beta-carotene, a compound found in carrots, helps protect vision, especially night vision.**

- Tomatoes provide vitamin C as well as vitamin K, biotin and B6. Vitamin B6 is indispensable to absorb magnesium properly. Lycopene, a powerful antioxidant found in tomatoes, is the "hot" antioxidant of the moment. Fresh tomatoes supply a fair amount of lycopene. But it is in cooked tomatoes and tomato sauce that you will find the highest level of cancer-fighting lycopene.

## Ingredients:

- 2 tomatoes
- 1 celery stalk
- 2 small carrots

## Directions:

-1- Rinse and pat dry all fruits/veggies. You can put your veggies directly in the juicer—no need to peel.
-2- Juice and drink right away, as antioxidants lose their potency as time passes.

Enjoy!

જી

# Sweet Dreams Red Boost

. For this drink, you will need your juicer.
. **The Sweet Dreams Red Boost provides several much-needed nutrients and phytochemicals:**
- **You will get your daily vitamin C recommended by the FDA, thanks to the apple, peach and strawberries in this drink.**
- Strawberries provide a high level of manganese and vitamin K, along with potent phenols (antioxidants), which make it an "anti-cancer" fruit.
- The peach will supply ample potassium, which new studies link to lower blood pressure.

## Ingredients:

- 1 peach
- 1 cup strawberries
- 2 small carrots
- 1 apple

## Directions:

**-1-** Rinse and pat dry all fruits/veggies. You can put your fruits/veggies directly in the juicer—no need to peel.
**-2-** Juice and drink right away, as antioxidants lose their potency as time passes.

Enjoy!

&

# Tomato Arugula Avocado Sandwich

This quick-to-make sandwich is a great, healthy way to get your vitamin E for the day, as avocado is the highest-ranking fruit source for vitamin E (yes, avocado is a fruit). **Also, avocados are one of the best sources of monounsaturated fat, the fat known to lower artery-clogging LDL cholesterol and raise heart-healthy HDL cholesterol.**
The tomatoes are a rich source of lycopene, a powerful antioxidant known to lower the risks of cancer and other degenerative diseases.

## Ingredients:

- 1 small avocado, peeled and divided
- ⅓ tablespoon lemon juice
- 1 tablespoon Dijon mustard
- ⅛ cup mayonnaise
- 2 slices whole-grain bread
- A handful of arugula
- 1 small tomato, sliced
- Salt and pepper to taste

## Directions:

-1- Process ½ the avocado, lemon juice, Dijon mustard and mayonnaise in a food processor until smooth.
-2- Spread this paste onto one slice of whole-grain bread.
-3- Top with tomato slices and arugula salad.
-4- Add salt and pepper to taste.
-5- Top with the sliced avocado half and sliced tomato.
-6- Cover with remaining slice of whole-grain bread.

Enjoy!

p.s. If you don't feel like having a sandwich, you can simply spread the avocado mix on each slice of bread and continue the topping process from there.

଼

# Arugula, Mushroom, and Raisin Salad

. **Because we cannot reproduce all antioxidants that can be found in vegetables in pill form, it is important to use a variety of different veggies in your salads. Dark-leafed arugula provides several potent antioxidants (as does spinach).**

. Mushrooms provide a high level of selenium, an essential mineral that works closely with vitamin E to produce antioxidants to neutralize the cell-damaging "free radicals" that can increase the risk of cancer and other age-related diseases. It plays an important role in the immune system, the thyroid system and the male reproductive system.

. Mushrooms also provide potassium and **copper**. Remember, iron and copper work together to create red blood cells.

. **Mushrooms also provide three vitamins from the B group; including riboflavin, which promotes healthy skin and good vision.**

. **Raisins provide phenols (powerful antioxidants) and are THE TOP SOURCE of the trace mineral boron. Boron is required to convert estrogen and vitamin D to their most active forms. Studies have shown that boron provides protection against osteoporosis.**

## Ingredients:

- 2 cups sliced button mushrooms
- 1 bunch arugula salad
- ½ cup raisins
- 1 tablespoon soyonnaise
- ½ cup chopped, dried tomatoes
- 4 thinly chopped basil leaves
- 2 tablespoons balsamic vinegar
- 1 tablespoon canola oil

## Directions:

-1- Put all the veggies and raisins in a large salad bowl.
-2- Drizzle oil and vinegar.
-3- Add soyonnaise.
-4- Mix.

Serves 4.

Enjoy!

∞

# Daily Fitness & Diet Log

Date

Overall Feeling Today:    ☺ ☹ ☹          Overall Fitness:          ☺ ☹ ☹
Overall Diet:             ☺ ☹ ☹          Overall Stress Level:     ☺ ☹ ☹

## Diet...

| Breakfast | Lunch | Dinner |
|---|---|---|
| _____ | _____ | _____ |
| _____ | _____ | _____ |
| _____ | _____ | _____ |
| _____ | _____ | _____ |
| _____ | _____ | _____ |

Extra meal (if any): _____

Fluid Intake: [        ] cups. Type of fluid: _____

Trans fats?... yes / no        Refined carbs?... yes / no        Home-made food?... yes / no

## Fitness...                                How many steps: [        ]

Flexibility      ☑☒: _____      ⊙: _____

MetaBoost        ☑☒: _____      ⊙: _____

Strength         ☑☒: _____      ⊙: _____

Cardio           ☑☒: _____      ⊙: _____

Other            ☑☒: _____      ⊙: _____

# Day 16: RED CLEANSE™

Get ready for a great cleanse. The RED CLEANSE™ will flush your system, while providing vitamins, minerals, antioxidants and other phytochemicals necessary for good health and proper nutrition.

Remember, you will need your juicer today. If you don't have a juicer, you can go to a juice bar today and order a juice made with the ingredients listed in the Red Cleanse™ recipes.

## EXERCISE DRILL—Day 16—Easy Walk

It is important that you do not overexert yourself today. **Go for three, 20-minute walks at a slow pace throughout the day.**

You may choose to do your 10-minute MetaBoost Exercise today and your 30-minute walk on an empty stomach, but if you do not have the energy to do so, please don't push yourself.

## NUTRITIONAL TIP—Day 16—Vitamin Facts

Vitamins and minerals are critical to good health and disease prevention. Fruits and vegetables are naturally full of these essential micronutrients, which are more easily absorbed into the bloodstream when consumed in juice form.

**The key players in the RED CLEANSE™ include vitamins A, C, K, and B6.** You will also consume plenty of lycopene, magnesium, potassium, beta-carotene, and other essential antioxidants, which prevent cell damage and, therefore, support immune system function, among other benefits.

**Vitamin A** improves weak eyesight, builds resistance to respiratory infections, and promotes healthy hair, skin, teeth and gums.

**Vitamin C** supports the immune system, is essential for connective tissue formation, and decreases blood cholesterol. Vitamin C is essential in the formation of collagen, which is found within the joint structure and keeps two bones from rubbing or bumping against one another. Lack of collagen leads to osteoarthritis, among other degenerative diseases.

**Vitamin K** is essential to building strong bones and preventing heart disease.

**Vitamin B6** is essential for the formation of red blood cells and blood antibodies. B6 is also critical for the absorption of magnesium.

**Can you see how they all work together?**

See you tomorrow,

*Valerie Your Private Coach*

# Daily Fitness & Diet Log

Date [ ]

Overall Feeling Today: ☺ ☺ ☹      Overall Fitness: ☺ ☺ ☹
Overall Diet: ☺ ☺ ☹     Overall Stress Level: ☺ ☺ ☹

## Diet...

| Breakfast | Lunch | Dinner |
|-----------|-------|--------|
| _____ | _____ | _____ |
| _____ | _____ | _____ |
| _____ | _____ | _____ |
| _____ | _____ | _____ |
| _____ | _____ | _____ |

Extra meal (if any): _____

Fluid Intake: [ ] cups. Type of fluid: _____

Trans fats?... yes / no    Refined carbs?... yes / no    Home-made food?... yes / no

## Fitness...

How many steps: [ ]

| | | | |
|-|-|-|-|
| Flexibility | ☑☒: _____ | ⏱: _____ |
| MetaBoost | ☑☒: _____ | ⏱: _____ |
| Strength | ☑☒: _____ | ⏱: _____ |
| Cardio | ☑☒: _____ | ⏱: _____ |
| Other | ☑☒: _____ | ⏱: _____ |

# Day 17: Training Camp (Days 17–21)

## Welcome to Training Camp!

How do you feel today after your cleanse yesterday? I hope you're feeling GREAT!

We are now back to our regular routine in terms of making your own healthy choices for breakfast, lunch, and dinner from your list of meal plans…But now we are into Training Camp, so things are going to be a little bit more challenging this week in terms of exercise. This is a BootCamp, after all!

**Along with your 30-minute daily walk, your 60-minutes of cumulative movement and your daily exercise drills, you will also perform MetaBoost #2 AT LEAST once per day (if not 2 or 3 times).** MetaBoost #2 is a 10-minute drill that will pump up your energy and give your metabolism a boost for hours after your workout.

Continue eating your healthy, balanced meals and following our daily exercise guidelines and drills, and you will be amazed with your results.

### EXERCISE DRILL—Day 17—Jumping Jacks

Keep that energy pumping! Along with your 30-minute walk on an empty stomach and your 10-minute MetaBoost, do 50 jumping jacks in the morning before eating breakfast. This will get your heart pumping and will boost your metabolism even more.

And remember to do 60 minutes of cumulative exercise every day, too.

# YOU CAN DO THIS!

## NUTRITIONAL TIP—Day 17—Salad Dressings

**Avoid store-bought salad dressings if at all possible.** Most store-bought salad dressings contain rancid fats that wreak havoc on your natural digestive system. They are unhealthy. Period.

For a healthy alternative, make your own dressing by mixing one table-spoon of olive oil with one tablespoon of balsamic vinegar or apple cider vinegar. Add a dab of Dijon mustard, and mix. Drizzle onto your salad sparingly (as usual) and enjoy.

See you tomorrow,

*Valerie Your Private Coach*

# Daily Fitness & Diet Log

Date

Overall Feeling Today:  ☺ ☺ ☹          Overall Fitness:          ☺ ☺ ☹
Overall Diet:           ☺ ☺ ☹          Overall Stress Level:    ☺ ☺ ☹

## Diet...

| Breakfast | Lunch | Dinner |
|-----------|-------|--------|
| _____ | _____ | _____ |
| _____ | _____ | _____ |
| _____ | _____ | _____ |
| _____ | _____ | _____ |
| _____ | _____ | _____ |

Extra meal (if any): _____

Fluid Intake: [          ] cups. Type of fluid: _____

Trans fats?... yes / no          Refined carbs?... yes / no          Home-made food?... yes / no

## Fitness...                    How many steps: [          ]

| Flexibility | ☑☒: _____ | ⊙: _____ |
| MetaBoost   | ☑☒: _____ | ⊙: _____ |
| Strength    | ☑☒: _____ | ⊙: _____ |
| Cardio      | ☑☒: _____ | ⊙: _____ |
| Other       | ☑☒: _____ | ⊙: _____ |

# Day 18: Training Camp
# (Days 17–21)

## How healthy is your heart?

Heart disease is one of the top killers in North America (the competition is always between heart disease and cancer). To prevent heart disease, you need to eat well and exercise—there's no secret here. Today we're REALLY going to get your heart pumping.

### EXERCISE DRILL—Day 18—Walk Uphill

To give yourself another boost in the cardiovascular department (which will help you build a healthy heart), **find somewhere where you can walk uphill today**.

Your heart is a muscle, and just like every other muscle, it needs to be exercised. Walking uphill requires more effort; therefore, more energy is expended and your heart works harder. You burn more calories and build stronger muscles in your back, glutes and legs, too. (Remember: building more lean muscle mass will increase your metabolism at rest, which means you will burn more calories throughout the day.) If you pump your arms and squeeze your abs, you are in for a total-body workout. And it doesn't take more than 30 minutes.

Be strong!

### NUTRITIONAL TIP—Day 18—The Five Joyful Rules of Eating

Today's tip is about mindful eating. Our bodies will tell us when we're hungry and will tell us when we're full. But far too often, we occupy ourselves with other activities while eating (driving, watching TV, sitting at the computer), which compromises our body's ability to tell us when to STOP EATING.

If you follow the Five Joyful Rules of Eating, you will be guaranteed to lose weight and maintain a healthy weight because your body will give you the signals you need to know when you've had enough. (Of course, it is up to you to listen to these signals.)

### The FIVE JOYFUL RULES OF EATING are...

**"Rule of Sitting"**—Sit down when you eat. Don't eat standing up or while walking. Sit down with a plate of food so that you know how much food you're putting into your mouth.

**"Rule of Awareness"**—When you eat, eat. Do not participate in a second activity (apart from enjoying your friends' company), no matter how convinced you are that you can do two things at once. Focus on the task at hand—eating—and become more aware of your body's signals.

**"Rule of Savor Each Bite"**—Be aware of what you're eating. Notice the texture of the food. Notice the flavors. Notice what your body is telling you about these foods. Feel the sensation of chewing, swallowing, and digesting. Let the flavors tantalize your taste buds.

**"Rule of One Bite"**—Chew and swallow one mouthful before taking another bite. SLOW DOWN when you eat.

**"Rule of Retreat"**—Relax when you eat. Allow your body to de-stress. Create joy in your eating environment, if at all possible. Play some music. Light some candles. Make eating a "no-stress" event; it will lead to better digestion and greater satisfaction.

Eat well and be well.

See you tomorrow,

*Valerie Your Private Coach*

# Daily Fitness & Diet Log

Date

| Overall Feeling Today: | ☺ ☺ ☹ | Overall Fitness: | ☺ ☺ ☹ |
| Overall Diet: | ☺ ☺ ☹ | Overall Stress Level: | ☺ ☺ ☹ |

## Diet...

| Breakfast | Lunch | Dinner |
| --- | --- | --- |
| _____ | _____ | _____ |
| _____ | _____ | _____ |
| _____ | _____ | _____ |
| _____ | _____ | _____ |
| _____ | _____ | _____ |

Extra meal (if any): _____

Fluid Intake: [          ] cups. Type of fluid: _____

Trans fats?... yes / no     Refined carbs?... yes / no     Home-made food?... yes / no

## Fitness...

How many steps: [          ]

| Flexibility | ☑☒: _____ | ⏲: _____ |
| MetaBoost | ☑☒: _____ | ⏲: _____ |
| Strength | ☑☒: _____ | ⏲: _____ |
| Cardio | ☑☒: _____ | ⏲: _____ |
| Other | ☑☒: _____ | ⏲: _____ |

# Day 19: Training Camp
# (Days 17–21)

Training Camp continues. Here we go…only 3 days left and then we'll move on to the fat-blaster portion of BootCamp.

## EXERCISE DRILL—Day 19—Sparring…
## Alone or with a Friend

**This is a great cardio boost…**

Stand with your feet shoulder-width apart and with your knees slightly bent facing your partner (but not too close) or a punching bag. Close your hands into fists. Choose an area in space on which to focus. Tighten your abs. Keep your hips facing forward as you punch straight forward (spar) into the air (or into a punching bag if you have one), repeatedly, one arm at a time.

Count 25 punches per side and then rest. **Punch as quickly as you can!** This works your heart, your arms, and your abdominals.

And, at the end of your quick punches, you can push your fists together **to work your biceps isometrically** (without movement). This will increase the strength in your arms. Push for at least 15 seconds, rest, and repeat. Be strong!

## NUTRITIONAL TIP—Day 19—Go Decaf

Replace your caffeinated beverages with decaffeinated ones.

**By choosing the decaffeinated varieties of your favorite beverages, you will decrease "the jitters" and your sleep pattern will return to normal, thereby helping you get a better night's sleep.**

And quality of sleep greatly effects productivity, awareness, and overall energy level.

From an antioxidant perspective, you can get the same benefits from decaf green tea as from regular green tea.

Recent studies have shown that **people with a regular sleep pattern tend to lose weight more easily** than those with an uneven sleep pattern. AND your blood levels of leptin, a hormone that acts as an appetite suppressant, appear to decrease when you experience sleep deprivation, according to new research. Keep leptin levels high and curb overeating and weight gain by getting at least 6 to 8 hours of sleep per night.

**Zzzzzzzzzzzzzzzz...**

See you tomorrow,

*Valerie Your Private Coach*

# Daily Fitness & Diet Log

Date

Overall Feeling Today:  ☺ ☻ ☹        Overall Fitness:        ☺ ☻ ☹
Overall Diet:           ☺ ☻ ☹        Overall Stress Level:   ☺ ☻ ☹

## Diet...

| Breakfast | Lunch | Dinner |
|-----------|-------|--------|
| _____ | _____ | _____ |
| _____ | _____ | _____ |
| _____ | _____ | _____ |
| _____ | _____ | _____ |
| _____ | _____ | _____ |

Extra meal (if any): _____

Fluid Intake: [        ] cups. Type of fluid: _____

Trans fats?... yes / no        Refined carbs?... yes / no        Home-made food?... yes / no

## Fitness...                              How many steps: [        ]

Flexibility      ☑☒: _____      🕐: _____

MetaBoost        ☑☒: _____      🕐: _____

Strength         ☑☒: _____      🕐: _____

Cardio           ☑☒: _____      🕐: _____

Other            ☑☒: _____      🕐: _____

# Day 20: Training Camp
# (Days 17–21)

**We're still going strong with Training Camp. Hang in there, you can do this!**

## EXERCISE DRILL—Day 20—Sprint

After your 30-minute walk this morning, find a 25-meter straight stretch (approximately the distance between two lamp posts) and **sprint the length of the stretch there and back** (50 meters total) as quickly as you can. Without stopping, jog there and back one more time, and then do one more sprint (there and back) before you cool down. A two-minute walk plus stretching is great for a cool down.

This is a fantastic workout from a cardiovascular perspective.

And if you find you need better running shoes, try the Nike Women's Shox TL or Nike Women's Air Alvord 2 and the Nike Men's Air Zoom Swift Vapor Trainer. I love those shoes. They are available at our on-line store at http://www.myprivatecoach.com/store.

Be strong!

## NUTRITIONAL TIP—Day 20—Water Alternative

If you crave sodas and/or sweet drinks, **stock your office and home with carbonated, unsweetened, flavored waters.**

The natural, fruity taste (make sure they are neither sweetened nor artificially sweetened) will help you satisfy your cravings without the sugar intake of regular sodas or the aspartame of diet sodas. Actually,

**carbonated, unsweetened, flavored waters contain ZERO sugar.** This is good news!

And even better, carbonated water counts towards your eight cups a day.

Now, go shopping. :o)

See you tomorrow,

*Valerie Your Private Coach*

# Daily Fitness & Diet Log

Date [                    ]

Overall Feeling Today: ☺ ☺ ☹     Overall Fitness: ☺ ☺ ☹
Overall Diet: ☺ ☺ ☹     Overall Stress Level: ☺ ☺ ☹

## Diet...

| Breakfast | Lunch | Dinner |
|-----------|-------|--------|
| _____ | _____ | _____ |
| _____ | _____ | _____ |
| _____ | _____ | _____ |
| _____ | _____ | _____ |
| _____ | _____ | |

Extra meal (if any): _____

Fluid Intake: [                ] cups. Type of fluid: _____

Trans fats?... yes / no     Refined carbs?... yes / no     Home-made food?... yes / no

## Fitness...          How many steps: [                ]

Flexibility   ☑☒: _____   ⏲: _____

MetaBoost   ☑☒: _____   ⏲: _____

Strength   ☑☒: _____   ⏲: _____

Cardio   ☑☒: _____   ⏲: _____

Other   ☑☒: _____   ⏲: _____

# Day 21: Training Camp
## (Days 17–21)

How are you feeling today? We're still going strong with Training Camp. Hang in there, you can do this!

### EXERCISE DRILL—Day 21—Side Kicks

**Side kicks are a great way to increase thigh strength and when done quickly, this exercise will also give you a great cardio boost.** Also, side kicks will help eliminate "saddlebags" if done as a cardio workout.

**Practice kicking techniques in front of a mirror.** This way, you can see what you are doing. For added balance and support, keep your hand against a wall while you are learning the technique.

Begin standing with feet shoulder-width apart. Keep your arms tight against your chest. Bring your right knee upward, and turn your knee and heel so that the bottom of your foot kicks out to the side. Extend the leg out to the side to strike with the bottom of the foot, and quickly retract the leg back to the right knee upward position. Return the leg and foot to the original standing position. While you are kicking, ensure that you bend the left knee for added balance. The left foot can pivot slightly for added strength. Repeat for opposite side.

The following key points should be remembered:

- Remain in control at all times. Do not use momentum too much or you will lose some benefits of this exercise. The slower you do your side kicks, the better. If you lack thigh strength, you may lose your balance. Kicking slowly and in control will help improve your strength and your overall balance.

- You can alternate fast kicks and slow kicks (five at a time, for instance) for variety and a greater challenge.
- Never overextend the kick. This adds pressure to the knee joint, and may also impair your balance.
- Always exhale when kicking. This increases the power of your technique.

Be strong!

## NUTRITIONAL TIP—Day 21—Avoid "Non-foods"

**Food is the most powerful drug you will ever take.** Non-foods not only provide empty calories for the body (calories that cannot be used for healthy body processes), but they actually DRAIN energy from your body, leaving you feeling sluggish and unmotivated.

**Avoid these energy-draining foods (non-foods) as much as possible, if not altogether.**

- White sugar
- White flour
- Pesticides and herbicides on conventional produce
- Conventional meat (which contains hormones, pesticides, herbicides)
- Most fast foods
- Deep-fried foods
- Rancid oils
- Trans fats

**Remember: one step in the right direction is worth a thousand years thinking about it.** Make one change at a time…soon, you will be eating healthier, will have more energy, and will be well on your way to a slimmer you.

See you tomorrow,

*Valerie Your Private Coach*

# Daily Fitness & Diet Log

Date [                    ]

Overall Feeling Today:  ☺ ☺ ☹        Overall Fitness:        ☺ ☺ ☹
Overall Diet:           ☺ ☺ ☹        Overall Stress Level:   ☺ ☺ ☹

## Diet...

Breakfast                Lunch                    Dinner

_____      _____      _____

_____      _____      _____

_____      _____      _____

_____      _____      _____

_____      _____      _____

Extra meal (if any): _____

Fluid Intake: [              ] cups. Type of fluid: _____

Trans fats?... yes / no      Refined carbs?... yes / no      Home-made food?... yes / no

## Fitness...                              How many steps: [              ]

Flexibility      ☑☒: _____      🕐: _____

MetaBoost        ☑☒: _____      🕐: _____

Strength         ☑☒: _____      🕐: _____

Cardio           ☑☒: _____      🕐: _____

Other            ☑☒: _____      🕐: _____

# Day 22: Fat-Blaster Camp (Days 22–28)

**It's already Week 4!**

Please **weigh yourself** and log your results in your **"Ultimate Daily Fitness and Diet Log"**. The Tanita Family Model Scale is perfect for this part of the BootCamp, since it easily calculates your body-fat percentage and weight at the same time. You can buy yours at: http://www.myprivatecoach.com/store.

## Welcome to the Fat-Blaster part of this program...

Contrary to popular belief, slow, anaerobic exercise does NOT promote fat loss UNLESS it is performed for long periods of time (longer than 60 minutes). For some people, this is good news. For others, not so good news. **The best way to REALLY get rid of unwanted fat in a short amount of time is to perform high-energy, cardiovascular activities.** It all comes down to calories (energy) burned. After all, to burn the highest number of calories in the shortest period of time, we need to exercise at a higher intensity and get our hearts pumping!

Interval training and quick sprints are the best way to promote healthy weight loss, so get ready for an intense, metabolism-boosting, fat-blasting week. You will receive MetaBoost Workout #3, which is to be incorporated into your Fat-Blaster Workout six days this week. Your instructions are below. (You can do this!)

**Along with the intense bouts of exercise, I will challenge you even further by requesting that you EAT A LIGHT DINNER EVERY NIGHT from the meal plans that you will receive this week, and from the meal plans you have already received.**

**Of course, whether or not you take this challenge is completely up to you.**

**Today's Goodies:**

- Breakfast, Lunch and Dinner Meal Plans for Days 22–28 (Rotate with the meal plans from Weeks 1, 2 and 3 for healthy variety. Remember to eat a LIGHT DINNER every night this week. Aren't choices wonderful?)
- Shopping List for Week 4
- MetaBoost Workout #3
- Dry Fig and Spinach Salad Recipe
- Peasant Lentil Soup Recipe
- Shrimp Avocado Recipe
- Daily Fitness & Diet Log

## FAT-BLASTER EXERCISE DRILL—Days 22–28

**For six out of the next seven days, you will need to follow this intense Fat-Blaster Exercise Routine:**

- Walk 30-minutes on an empty stomach (as usual).
- Complete MetaBoost Workout #3 (15 minutes).
- Do 120 crunches, fast (resting every 30 crunches); this should not take more than 4 minutes.
- In the afternoon or before dinner, do another MetaBoost Workout (#1, #2 or #3)—preferably MetaBoost Workout #3. Doing the MetaBoost Workout before dinner raises the natural level of endorphins in your body, thereby decreasing your appetite.

On your rest day, when you do not do the Fat Blaster Exercise Routine, be sure to continue with your 30-minute walk (EVERY DAY), 60 minutes of cumulative exercise, and one MetaBoost Workout (#1, #2 or #3).

Be strong!

## NUTRITIONAL TIP—Day 22—How about using Metabolism-Boosting Pills instead of doing my workout?

**How tempting! You can spend $99 or even less, and without changing your lifestyle and without exercising, you can get rid of those extra pounds…**

Based on the latest figures, Americans spend a staggering $30 to $50 billion a year on dieting, $6 billion of which are spent on diet products, pills, patches and methods which are fraudulent *(in "Fat—Exploding the Myths"—Lisa Colles-).* A fraudulent product can range from being totally ineffective to having dramatic health consequences (even death).

**Needless to say, never, ever, ever buy or ingest ANY diet pill (unless prescribed by a doctor).**

We can certainly divide diet pills into two types: prescription-only diet pills and over-the-counter (OTC) diet pills. Doctors who believe that emergency weight loss is vital may prescribe prescription-only pills to severely obese patients. In this case, the pills act as a quick, necessary fix, but will never replace the importance of developing a healthy lifestyle with a balanced fitness routine.

For those who are not considered morbidly obese by their doctors (and hence, should not require diet pills), there are OTC diet pills. Because these pills are NOT regulated by the FDA (they are classified as food supplements instead of drugs), **manufacturers make unverifiable claims and these pills can have deadly effects. The words "natural," "herbal" and "organic" should not lure you into thinking that these products are safe and effective. Most of them AREN'T!**

Keep in mind that **the vast majority of metabolism-boosting pills contain ingredients that artificially increase your heart rate, which can lead to fatal heart attacks.** One such ingredient is ephedrine, which has been linked to several deaths already.

So what about diet patches? There may be less danger (physiologically) in using diet patches, but they are completely ineffective. It has been shown that dieters on the patch tend to overeat, because they think that the patch will take care of their excess calorie intake. This DOESN'T HAPPEN!

And besides, **wearing a patch will never transform an unhealthy lifestyle into a healthy one.**

**AGAIN, YOU DO NOT NEED DIET PILLS OR PATCHES TO LOSE WEIGHT.** They are unhealthy and potentially dangerous. The key to permanent weight loss is a gradual, healthy lifestyle change.

See you tomorrow,

*Valerie Your Private Coach*

# Meal Suggestions—Days 22 to 28

# Mix & Match

## ❀ Breakfast

| Choice #1 | Choice #2 | Choice #3—Light |
|---|---|---|
| Two-egg veggie omelet | Slow-cooked oatmeal | 2 slices of whole-grain bread, 2 tablespoons non-hydrogenated margarine |
| slice of whole-grain bread | 2 tablespoons plain yogurt, Stevia | 2 slices smoked salmon |
| 1 cup of berries | A few berries | ½ grapefruit |

## ❀ Lunch

| Choice #1 - Middle-Eastern | Choice #2 | Choice #3 - Light |
|---|---|---|
| *Shrimp Avocado* | Grilled turkey patty | *Dry Fig and Spinach Salad* |
| Israeli salad | Steamed butter beans sprinkled with paprika 1 slice of whole-grain bread | 2 slices of whole-grain bread |
| 1 apple | | A few berries |

## ❀ Dinner

| Choice #1—Japanese | Choice #2 | Choice #3—Quick |
|---|---|---|
| Green salad with dressing Miso soup | *Peasant Lentil Soup* 1 slice of whole-grain bread | Campbell's Select Soup Spinach salad |
| Yakitori or sashimi | 1 pear | 1 frozen fruit bar |

# ഔ **Shopping List—Week 4** ഔ

| Vegetables, Legumes & Nuts | Fruit |
|---|---|
| - ½ pound butter beans<br>- 3 bunches fresh spinach<br>- Raw, dry pumpkin seeds (optional)<br>- 1 shallot<br>- 200 grams green lentils<br>- 2 carrots<br>- 1 celery stalk<br>- 2 onions<br>- 2 tomatoes<br>- 1 clove of garlic<br>- 1 laurel leaf + thyme<br>- 1 tablespoon oregano<br>- 1 tablespoon minced basil<br>- 2 tablespoon minced parsley<br>- Campbell's Select Soup<br>- 2 avocados | - 3 cups of berries (your choice)<br>- 1 grapefruit<br>- 10 dry figs<br>- 1 pear |

| Eggs & Dairy | Meat, Fish & Tofu |
|---|---|
| - 2 eggs<br>- 1 plain yogurt | - 1 turkey patty<br>- 150 grams thin bacon or low-fat prosciutto<br>- 200 grams Serrano ham or prosciutto<br>- 500 grams shrimp |

| Oils & Sweets | Miscellaneous |
|---|---|
| - Olive oil<br>- Canola oil<br>- Canola oil spray | - Whole-grain bread (small loaf)<br>- Slow-cooked oatmeal<br>- 1 small package wild salmon<br>- Paprika<br>- Wine vinegar<br>- Frozen fruit bar |

# MetaBoost Workout #3 (15-Minute Drill)

For those of us who are pressed for time, there is always a way to squeeze in exercise, every single day.

It is important that you fit cardio, strength, flexibility, body alignment and de-stress training into your routine as often as possible.

This 15-minute, metabolism-boosting workout has been created specifically for you. You can perform this routine several times throughout your day. The more often you move the better. This workout will help you boost your metabolism, which is what you need in order to lose weight for good.

## 15-Minute MetaBoost

1 min march in place (warm up)
20 jumping jacks
20 side to side leaps
1 min push-ups
1 min abs (you choose)
1 min march in place
20 jumping jacks
20 side to side leaps
1 min abs
1 min squats
4-min power walk
2 min lunges
1-min sun breath: standing, inhale and raise your arms overhead. Exhale and fold forward at hips.

# Dry Fig Spinach Salad

This dish is an excellent source of vitamin C and calcium.
. Spinach is a rich source of powerful antioxidants and calcium.
. Dried figs are in the Top Five when it comes to the best food sources of calcium.
. Shallots are also loaded with vitamin C.

## Ingredients:

- 2 bunches of fresh spinach (the fresher the better)
- 10 dry figs cut into quarters
- 2 tablespoons canola oil
- 1 tablespoon balsamic vinegar
- Dry pumpkin seeds (optional)
- 1 tablespoon Dijon mustard
- 2 tablespoons minced shallots
- Salt and pepper to taste

## Directions:

-1- Prepare the vinaigrette in a small bowl; mix (with a fork) mustard, vinegar, minced shallots and salt and pepper (to taste). The best thing to do is to wait for 10–15 minutes so that the shallots are infused with the balsamic vinegar.
-2- Wash, spin and cut spinach leaves. Put in a salad bowl with dry figs and seeds. Mix and refrigerate.
-3- Add oil to vinaigrette. Mix.
-4- Just before serving, add vinaigrette to spinach, figs, and seeds and mix.

Enjoy!

Serves 4.

## Variations:

To reduce the glycemic index of this recipe, you can replace the figs with dried apricots.

∞

# Peasant Lentil Soup

. Lentils and beans have been eaten for thousands of years. They are believed to have originated in the Middle East.
. Lentils are a great source of fiber and complex carbohydrates. They are also extremely low in fat, making them an ideal staple for any diet. For those of us who don't eat enough animal protein, lentils are an excellent vegetable protein source.
. Lentils are also a good source of vitamin B5, a vitamin needed to manufacture adrenal hormones and chemicals that regulate nerve functions.
. Lentils also provide phosphorus, a necessary companion of calcium for building bones and teeth. Furthermore, lentils and beans absorb flavors more than the average veggie, which makes for fun and tasty dishes.
. **You can double the ingredients and freeze (in individual portions) this wonderful soup. When you are in a hurry, just unfreeze one portion.**

## Ingredients:

- 200 grams green lentils
- 150 grams thin bacon or low-fat prosciutto
- 200 grams Serrano ham or prosciutto
- 2 carrots
- 1 celery stalk
- 2 onions
- 2 tomatoes
- 1 garlic clove
- 1 laurel leaf + thyme
- 1 tablespoon oregano
- 1 tablespoon minced basil
- 2 tablespoons minced parsley
- 2 tablespoons olive oil
- 2 tablespoons wine vinegar
- Salt and pepper to taste

## Directions:

-1- Cover lentils with cold water. Bring to a boil. Boil for 3 minutes, then drain.
-2- In a large pot, sauté sliced onions in olive oil for 3 minutes.
-3- Add bacon, ham/prosciutto and all veggies, peeled and cut in small pieces.
-4- Simmer for 5 minutes and add lentils, 1½ liters of cold water, laurel leaf, thyme, mashed garlic and oregano.
-5- Add pepper and salt (remember: ham is naturally salty, so don't over-salt).
-6- Cover and simmer for 1 hour.

**-7-** After 1 hour, remove laurel leaf and thyme. Add vinegar.
**-8-** Add pepper and salt, if necessary, and sprinkle parsley and basil on top right before serving.

Enjoy!

Serves 8.

ଛଓ

# Shrimp Avocado

. This very quick-to-make recipe is a great, healthy way to get your vitamin E for the day, as avocado is the highest-ranking fruit source for vitamin E (yes, avocado is a fruit).
. **Also, avocados are one of the best sources of monounsaturated fat, the fat known to lower artery-clogging LDL cholesterol and raise heart-healthy HDL cholesterol.**
. Shrimp is a good source of copper, zinc and selenium. Zinc is a necessary element in more than 100 enzymes that are essential for digestion and metabolism, while selenium is a powerful antioxidant.

## Ingredients:

- 1 small avocado, divided
- ½ cup cooked and peeled shrimp
- ⅓ tablespoon lemon juice
- ⅛ cup soyonnaise
- 1 small tomato, diced
- Salt and pepper to taste

## Directions:

-1- In a bowl, mix shrimp, soyonnaise, lemon juice, diced tomatoes, and salt and pepper.
-2- Fill each side of the avocado with mix.
-3- For decoration purposes, you can sprinkle some minced parsley.

೮ა

# Daily Fitness & Diet Log

Date [          ]

Overall Feeling Today: ☺ ☻ ☹          Overall Fitness: ☺ ☻ ☹
Overall Diet: ☺ ☻ ☹          Overall Stress Level: ☺ ☻ ☹

## Diet...

| Breakfast | Lunch | Dinner |
|---|---|---|
| _____ | _____ | _____ |
| _____ | _____ | _____ |
| _____ | _____ | _____ |
| _____ | _____ | _____ |
| _____ | _____ | _____ |

Extra meal (if any): _____

Fluid Intake: [          ] cups. Type of fluid: _____

Trans fats?... yes / no          Refined carbs?... yes / no          Home-made food?... yes / no

## Fitness...          How many steps: [          ]

Flexibility          ☑☒: _____          🕐: _____

MetaBoost          ☑☒: _____          🕐: _____

Strength          ☑☒: _____          🕐: _____

Cardio          ☑☒: _____          🕐: _____

Other          ☑☒: _____          🕐: _____

# Day 23: Fat-Blaster Camp (Days 22–28)

How was your first day of the Fat-Blaster workout? I am sure you got your heart pumping with that routine.

Remember, it is important to move at your own pace, but at the same time, in order to see RESULTS, you will need to **push yourself beyond your normal comfort zone.** If the exercises are too easy, they won't elicit much change.

## EXERCISE DRILL—Day 23—Fat-Blaster Day 2

Continue with the Fat-Blaster Workout:

- Walk 30-minutes on an empty stomach (as usual).
- Complete MetaBoost Workout #3 (15 minutes).
- Do 120 crunches, fast (resting every 30 crunches); this should not take more than 4 minutes.
- In the afternoon or before dinner, do another MetaBoost Workout (#1, #2 or #3)—preferably MetaBoost Workout #3.

Think about contracting your abdominals throughout the routine—especially while walking.

Be strong!

## NUTRITIONAL TIP—Day 23—What to Eat/Drink After a Really Hard Workout...

Are you ready for this one?

After a hard workout, the most basic (and best) thing to do is to **DRINK WATER AND ONLY WATER.**

The body needs to replenish its water stores since so much water is released as sweat while exercising.

No food is absolute necessary right away unless you are about to begin a very intense activity soon after your workout (construction work, lifting heavy lumber, etc.) or an activity where you might not have access to food for a while (a long trip to the beach, for example).

In these cases, a low glycemic meal would be great, as it will not send your blood sugar through the roof; and, therefore, you will store less energy as fat at your next meal.

*Here are some great post-workout mini-meals:*

- Hummus + whole-wheat pita bread
- Plain yogurt
- Kefir + Stevia
- A cup of strawberries + 1 slice of whole-grain bread + 1 teaspoon of low-fat cream cheese.

**In any case, you DO NOT HAVE to eat after a workout. Just drink lots and lots of water!**

Have a great workout today!

*Valerie Your Private Coach*

# Daily Fitness & Diet Log

Date [                    ]

Overall Feeling Today: ☺ ☺ ☹      Overall Fitness: ☺ ☺ ☹
Overall Diet: ☺ ☺ ☹      Overall Stress Level: ☺ ☺ ☹

## Diet...

| Breakfast | Lunch | Dinner |
| --- | --- | --- |
| _____ | _____ | _____ |
| _____ | _____ | _____ |
| _____ | _____ | _____ |
| _____ | _____ | _____ |
| _____ | _____ | _____ |

Extra meal (if any): _____

Fluid Intake: [            ] cups. Type of fluid: _____

Trans fats?... yes / no      Refined carbs?... yes / no      Home-made food?... yes / no

## Fitness...                          How many steps: [            ]

Flexibility        ☑☒: _____    ⏱: _____

MetaBoost        ☑☒: _____    ⏱: _____

Strength        ☑☒: _____    ⏱: _____

Cardio        ☑☒: _____    ⏱: _____

Other        ☑☒: _____    ⏱: _____

# Day 24: Fat-Blaster Camp
# (Days 22–28)

Have you ever had one of those days when you just didn't feel like exercising? I have those days, too. And even though it sounds a bit "cliché," if you just get moving, you will likely end up enjoying your workout.

**Exercise actually gives you energy because of the release of endorphins (endorphins are natural biochemical substances produced by the human nervous system that elevate mood and/or kill pain). And when you feel good, you have more energy, right?**

### EXERCISE DRILL—Day 24—Fat-Blaster Day 3

Continue with the Fat-Blaster Workout:

- Walk 30-minutes on an empty stomach (as usual).
- Complete MetaBoost Workout #3 (15 minutes).
- Do 120 crunches, fast (resting every 30 crunches); this should not take more than 4 minutes.
- In the afternoon or before dinner, do another MetaBoost Workout (#1, #2 or #3)—preferably MetaBoost Workout #3.

Think about each muscle you are using while working out. **Just thinking about the muscle will increase its resistance by up to 10%!** This is what scientists call the "mind-body connection." It's very powerful.

Be strong!

## NUTRITIONAL TIP—Day 24—Fabulous Figs

Whether you savor flavorful figs as a snack or in your favorite recipes, **figs are rich in complex carbohydrates (the body's main source of energy), are an excellent source of dietary fiber, and contain a wealth of essential minerals, including calcium, iron, and potassium.**

**Did you know that a half-cup of figs contains as much calcium as a half-cup of milk?** It's true! Although the natural sugar content in fruits is higher than in vegetables, enjoying four chewy, flavorful figs will give you the calcium you need for strong teeth and bones, without having to consume dairy products.

Many people do not get their recommended daily intake of calcium, and those especially at risk of not consuming enough calcium are women and growing teens.

Try our "Dry Fig Spinach Salad Recipe" for a delicious, calcium-rich meal.

**p.s. To avoid the blood-sugar surge, try eating a half cup of low-fat kefir before you eat your figs.** Kefir is a cultured, enzyme-rich food filled with friendly micro-organisms that help balance your "inner ecosystem." More nutritious and therapeutic than yogurt, it supplies complete protein, essential minerals, and valuable B vitamins. It also contributes to a healthy immune system. You can buy kefir at most health food stores.

Bon Appétit,

*Valerie Your Private Coach*

# Daily Fitness & Diet Log

Date

Overall Feeling Today: ☺ ☺ ☹        Overall Fitness:        ☺ ☺ ☹
Overall Diet:          ☺ ☺ ☹        Overall Stress Level:  ☺ ☺ ☹

## Diet...

| Breakfast | Lunch | Dinner |
|-----------|-------|--------|
| _____ | _____ | _____ |
| _____ | _____ | _____ |
| _____ | _____ | _____ |
| _____ | _____ | _____ |
| _____ | _____ | _____ |

Extra meal (if any): _____

Fluid Intake: [          ] cups. Type of fluid: _____

Trans fats?... yes / no        Refined carbs?... yes / no        Home-made food?... yes / no

## Fitness...                    How many steps: [          ]

Flexibility      ☑☒: _____      🕐: _____

MetaBoost        ☑☒: _____      🕐: _____

Strength         ☑☒: _____      🕐: _____

Cardio           ☑☒: _____      🕐: _____

Other            ☑☒: _____      🕐: _____

# Day 25: Fat-Blaster Camp
# (Days 22–28)

Only 5 more days to go! You're doing GREAT!

What are the changes you have seen in your energy level so far? What healthy habits have you developed, and which ones still need some practice?

Take a look at your successes each day and **acknowledge yourself for what you ARE doing first…**and then take a look at areas where you can improve your performance. There are some challenging parts to this program, but you know your "why" and you know what it takes to achieve your dream weight, so you can and will have it all. Ask yourself: What needs to happen today to finish this program as a winner?

Keep going…And have a wonderful day!

## EXERCISE DRILL—Day 25—Fat Blaster Day 4

Continue with the Fat-Blaster Workout:

- Walk 30-minutes on an empty stomach (as usual).
- Complete MetaBoost Workout #3 (15 minutes).
- Do 120 crunches, fast (resting every 30 crunches); this should not take more than 4 minutes.
- In the afternoon or before dinner, do another MetaBoost Workout (#1, #2 or #3)—preferably MetaBoost Workout #3.

**Why do the crunches fast?** Although many people (including your favorite personal trainer) believe that crunches must be done slowly to elicit the best results, doing your crunches quickly actually puts the muscle in an anaerobic state (you can feel the "burn" due to the lactic acid build-up). Anaerobic exercise uses fat as its energy source.

Trust us on this one…**When you do your crunches quickly and in high quantity—120 to 200 at a time- you will create a flat stomach in no time** as long as you are reducing your body fat at the same time (which you are doing with the combination of cardiovascular exercise and healthy, balanced meal plans).

Be strong!

## NUTRITIONAL TIP—Day 25—Food Labels

Every person should understand how food labels work, but most people have been misled when it comes to understanding how to read them. **Here are some helpful tips to help you wisely determine the fat content in foods:**

**-1-** Understand that 1 gram of carbohydrate or protein will give you 4 calories of energy. 1 gram of fat will give you 9 calories of energy.

**-2-** Your diet should contain NO MORE than 30% of its daily calories from fat.

**-3-** To find out at a glance if a product meets that criteria, look at the total fat grams in a serving, and multiply that number by 9 to get the total number of calories from fat. Then, divide your answer by the total number of calories in a serving size and multiply by 100. Now you know what the percentage of fat is in your product.

For example, a serving of bran cereal (30g) contains approximately 75 calories and 1 gram of fat. 1 gram of fat times 9 calories per fat gram = 9 calories from fat. 9 calories from fat divided by 75 calories per serving = 0.12 times 100 = 12%. (It's okay if you need your calculator at first.) So this food is 12% fat.

How about products that claim to be fat-free, like many non-stick cooking sprays?

1 serving (spray) of a leading non-stick cooking spray contains 4 calories and 0.4 grams of fat. 0.4 times 9 calories per fat gram = 3.6 calories from fat. If a total serving is 4 calories, and in one serving you get

3.6 calories from fat, you can see that this is nearly a 100% fat food, even though the label on the front says fat-free!

Be careful!

Not all fat is bad, in fact, **you need fat to live. Good fats are unsaturated fats like olive oil, canola oil, and safflower oil, and the fats found in nuts, seeds and avocados.**

By knowing this simple equation, you can pick up a product quickly at the grocery store and decide whether or not it meets your criteria for health. **Remember, if it is more than 30% fat, think twice.** Or make sure that most of your foods are lower in fat to make up for a splurge every now and again.

p.s. Remember to only eat a LIGHT dinner tonight.

Until tomorrow…Enjoy the sunshine,

*Valerie Your Private Coach*

# Daily Fitness & Diet Log

Date [                    ]

Overall Feeling Today: ☺ ☺ ☹     Overall Fitness: ☺ ☺ ☹
Overall Diet: ☺ ☺ ☹             Overall Stress Level: ☺ ☺ ☹

## Diet...

| Breakfast | Lunch | Dinner |
| --- | --- | --- |
| _____ | _____ | _____ |
| _____ | _____ | _____ |
| _____ | _____ | _____ |
| _____ | _____ | _____ |
| _____ | _____ | _____ |

Extra meal (if any): _____

Fluid Intake: [            ] cups. Type of fluid: _____

Trans fats?... yes / no     Refined carbs?... yes / no     Home-made food?... yes / no

## Fitness...                       How many steps: [            ]

Flexibility     ☑☒: _____ ⏰: _____

MetaBoost       ☑☒: _____ ⏰: _____

Strength        ☑☒: _____ ⏰: _____

Cardio          ☑☒: _____ ⏰: _____

Other           ☑☒: _____ ⏰: _____

# Day 26: Fat-Blaster Camp
# (Days 22–28)

Only 4 more days to go!

**Visualize yourself thin.** I know this might sound a bit strange, but one of the things I know for sure is that our minds will sabotage anything that doesn't feel real or "safe" for us. So, if you have always seen yourself as a heavy person, when you start shedding those extra pounds, your mind won't recognize you and may try to take you off track by giving you a million-and-one excuses as to why you cannot lose the extra weight.

**Your mind cannot distinguish between something real or imagined**, so if you visualize yourself thin, you will have a higher likelihood that your mind will accept the new you, and help you maintain your new, healthy weight.

And if you really want to see and experience great results—fast—**light a candle and watch the candle burning as you visualize your new, slim self, and feel what it would feel like to live and walk in a leaner body.**

Visualizing yourself thin for 2–3 minutes every morning and evening should be enough to do the trick.

## EXERCISE DRILL—Day 26—Fat Blaster Day 5

## Go, Go, Go!

**Continue with the Fat-Blaster Workout today:**

- Walk 30-minutes on an empty stomach (as usual).
- Complete MetaBoost Workout #3 (15 minutes).

- Do 120 crunches, fast (resting every 30 crunches); this should not take more than 4 minutes.
- In the afternoon or before dinner, do another MetaBoost Workout (#1, #2 or #3)—preferably MetaBoost Workout #3.

Remember, as you do your exercises, visualize the muscles moving (mind-body connection) and **see yourself in the shape you want to achieve**. You will greatly enhance your likelihood of life-long success. Be strong!

## NUTRITIONAL TIP—Day 26—The Importance of Calcium

Minerals are body-building elements that also aid in specific body functions including digestion and temperature regulation. One of the major essential minerals is calcium.

Calcium is required for bone and tooth formation, blood clotting, muscle contraction and nerve transmission. **Make sure you consume between 1,000–1,200 mg of calcium per day (more if you are a pregnant or post-menopausal woman, or a teen).** Dark, green, leafy vegetables, sea vegetables, nuts, legumes, sardines, figs, low-fat dairy and other calcium-enriched foods will all contribute to a healthy, calcium-rich diet.

See you tomorrow,

*Valerie Your Private Coach*

# Daily Fitness & Diet Log

Date

Overall Feeling Today: ☺ ☺ ☹          Overall Fitness:          ☺ ☺ ☹
Overall Diet: ☺ ☺ ☹                        Overall Stress Level:   ☺ ☺ ☹

## Diet...

| Breakfast | Lunch | Dinner |
|-----------|-------|--------|
| _____ | _____ | _____ |
| _____ | _____ | _____ |
| _____ | _____ | _____ |
| _____ | _____ | _____ |
| _____ | _____ | _____ |

Extra meal (if any): _____

Fluid Intake: [        ] cups. Type of fluid: _____

Trans fats?... yes / no       Refined carbs?... yes / no       Home-made food?... yes / no

## Fitness...                                       How many steps: [        ]

Flexibility        ☑☒: _____        🕐: _____

MetaBoost        ☑☒: _____        🕐: _____

Strength          ☑☒: _____        🕐: _____

Cardio             ☑☒: _____        🕐: _____

Other               ☑☒: _____        🕐: _____

# Day 27: Fat-Blaster Camp (Days 22–28)

### Only 3 days left in the 30-day BootCamp!

Remember to do your 3 sets of 100 glute contractions today and at least 3 sets of 20 push-ups against any wall. The great thing about these exercises is that they can be done ANYWHERE. **The more activity you fit into your everyday life, the more likely you will keep the weight off, for good, thanks to the lean muscle mass you will build. Having more lean muscle will help boost your metabolism, so that you burn more calories even at rest.**

No sense going back to old habits now!

Sure, developing these new habits takes practice, but the results are well worth it.

## EXERCISE DRILL—Day 27—Fat Blaster Day 6

All right, keep up the pace and continue with the Fat-Blaster Workout today:

- Walk 30-minutes on an empty stomach (as usual).
- Complete MetaBoost Workout #3 (15 minutes).
- Do 120 crunches, fast (resting every 30 crunches); this should not take more than 4 minutes.
- In the afternoon or before dinner, do another MetaBoost Workout (#1, #2 or #3)—preferably MetaBoost Workout #3.

You may choose to do your glute contractions while walking today and you can stop mid-way and do a set or two of wall push-ups, too. Might as well get it all in at once.

Be strong!

## NUTRITIONAL TIP—Day 27—Cook for yourself

Besides tasting better and being healthier for you, **cooking your own meals actually prevents over-eating due to the pure enjoyment of tasting your food.** Baking your own bread or simmering your own soups is a wonderful reason to slow down, chew your food, and smell the aroma...Mmmmmm...

See you tomorrow,

*Valerie Your Private Coach*

# Daily Fitness & Diet Log

Date [            ]

Overall Feeling Today:   ☺ ☺ ☹        Overall Fitness:        ☺ ☺ ☹
Overall Diet:            ☺ ☺ ☹        Overall Stress Level:   ☺ ☺ ☹

## Diet...

| Breakfast | Lunch | Dinner |
|-----------|-------|--------|
| _____ | _____ | _____ |
| _____ | _____ | _____ |
| _____ | _____ | _____ |
| _____ | _____ | _____ |
| _____ | _____ | _____ |

Extra meal (if any): _____

Fluid Intake: [            ] cups. Type of fluid: _____

Trans fats?... yes / no        Refined carbs?... yes / no        Home-made food?... yes / no

## Fitness...                          How many steps: [            ]

Flexibility      ☑☒: _____    ◷: _____

MetaBoost        ☑☒: _____    ◷: _____

Strength         ☑☒: _____    ◷: _____

Cardio           ☑☒: _____    ◷: _____

Other            ☑☒: _____    ◷: _____

# Day 28: Fat-Blaster Camp
# (Days 22–28)

**Only 2 days left. Let's GO!**

Take a look at your results so far in your **"Ultimate Daily Fitness and Diet Log."** How are you doing? You should be seeing incredible progress. Have your results surprised you?

To maintain your weight, rather than continue losing weight, be sure to increase your portion sizes (just a little bit) or to include one or two healthy snacks (from your Snack List) to your daily diet. I prefer eliminating snacks altogether, but everyone is different and only you know what is best for you.

## EXERCISE DRILL—Day 28—Fat Blaster Day 7

Give yourself a real push today:

- Walk 30-minutes on an empty stomach (as usual).
- Complete MetaBoost Workout #3 (15 minutes).
- Do 120 crunches, fast (resting every 30 crunches); this should not take more than 4 minutes.
- In the afternoon or before dinner, do another MetaBoost Workout (#1, #2 or #3)—preferably MetaBoost Workout #3.

Push, push, push! Make it count!

Be strong!

## NUTRITIONAL TIP—Day 28—Tummy ache?

Though not supported by long-term, double-blind studies, empirical observations have shown that mint herbal tea (just hot water and mint leaves) helps keep your stomach flat by reducing acid buildup and improving digestion.

Simply take 10 fresh mint leaves, and let them steep in hot water for 3–4 minutes. Enjoy after any meal or even between meals. It's that simple.

See you tomorrow,

*Valerie Your Private Coach*

# Daily Fitness & Diet Log

Date _____

| | | | |
|---|---|---|---|
| Overall Feeling Today: | ☺ ☺ ☹ | Overall Fitness: | ☺ ☺ ☹ |
| Overall Diet: | ☺ ☺ ☹ | Overall Stress Level: | ☺ ☺ ☹ |

## Diet...

| Breakfast | Lunch | Dinner |
|---|---|---|
| _____ | _____ | _____ |
| _____ | _____ | _____ |
| _____ | _____ | _____ |
| _____ | _____ | _____ |
| _____ | _____ | _____ |

Extra meal (if any): _____

Fluid Intake: _____ cups. Type of fluid: _____

Trans fats?... yes / no          Refined carbs?... yes / no          Home-made food?... yes / no

## Fitness...                    How many steps: _____

| | | |
|---|---|---|
| Flexibility | ☑☒: _____ | ◷: _____ |
| MetaBoost | ☑☒: _____ | ◷: _____ |
| Strength | ☑☒: _____ | ◷: _____ |
| Cardio | ☑☒: _____ | ◷: _____ |
| Other | ☑☒: _____ | ◷: _____ |

# Day 29: BONUS DRILL
# (Days 29 & 30)

## You've come a long way!

Four weeks of healthy eating and intense movement: I hope you are happy with your results.

Most crash diets are ridiculous at best and dangerous at worst. I normally do not recommend crash diets to our clients, but if you're going to go on a crash diet anyway, you might as well eat nutritious foods, and take care of your body, mind and soul throughout the process.

*Remember, if you continue eating a nutritionally balanced diet, such as this one, with daily movement and other muscle-building activities, you will continue to lose weight and/or maintain your goal weight. This entire program is about making healthy CHOICES, not restricting your diet for the rest of your life. Hopefully, you have learned many of the tricks to keep the weight off, and to continue improving your fitness level as well.*

**Go, Go, Go!**

**Bonus Drill Goodies:**

- MetaBoost Workout #4 BONUS (12-minute drill)
- Avocado Sandwich Recipe
- Goat Cheese and Berries Salad Recipe
- Braised Cabbage Recipe
- Healthy Pizza Recipe
- Grilled Stilton Patty Recipe
- Daily Fitness & Diet Log

## EXERCISE DRILL—Day 29—BE CREATIVE

Okay, you have spent 4 weeks walking every morning, doing your MetaBoost exercises, following helpful tips and strategies to make your exercise more effective. **So now it's your turn to take responsibility for your daily exercise and overall fitness. You can do this!**

We highly recommend that you continue walking for 30 minutes every morning on an empty stomach, and continue getting at least 60 minutes of cumulative exercise daily (as per the Surgeon General's recommendations). Since you have been doing this for four weeks, you have had enough time to develop this healthy, lifestyle habit. Continue using it to ensure that the weight you have lost stays off for good.

And be sure to do at least one MetaBoost workout per day. Be strong!

## NUTRITIONAL TIP—Day 29—VARIETY

Did you know that today's global population relies on fewer than 20 staples, including wheat, maize, rice, barley and oats?

Our ancient ancestors consumed thousands of different roots, grains, nuts, leafy plants, grass seeds, fruits, stalks, tubers, gums and flowers. Nowadays, potatoes are the only staple root crop on most North American farms. We eat mainly domesticated meats with little variety, compared to the hundreds of species of wild game in our ancestors' diet. Did you know that more than 12,000 hamburgers are consumed across the United States EVERY MINUTE? Incredible.

If you do enjoy eating meat, choose wild game over domesticated meats as often as possible. Wild game has a very, very low level of fat, including saturated fat. Here is a list of suppliers of wild game meats, for your reference:

www.brokenarrowranch.com (check out their nutrition data page and compare the nutritional value of beef to antelope…)
www.hillsfoods.com (This one is in BC, Canada…and they have frogs, too.)
www.americangourmet.net

And tomorrow we cross the finish line...

*Valerie Your Private Coach*

# MetaBoost Workout #4 (12-Minute Drill)

For those of us who are pressed for time, there is always a way to squeeze in exercise, every single day.

It is important that you fit cardio, strength, flexibility, body alignment and de-stress training into your routine as often as possible.

This 12-minute, metabolism-boosting workout has been created specifically for you. You can perform this routine several times throughout your day. The more often you move the better. This workout will help you boost your metabolism, which is what you need in order to lose weight for good.

---

### 12-Minute MetaBoost

1 min march in place (warm up)
2-min power walk
1 min squats
1 min lunges
1 min march in place
1 min abdominal crunches
1 min side abs
1-min power walk
1 min push-ups
2-min sun breath: standing, inhale and raise your arms overhead. Exhale, keep your legs straight, and bend forward at hips. Feel the stretch. Repeat 4 times.

---

# Avocado Sandwich

. This quick-to-make sandwich is a great, healthy way to get your vitamin E for the day, as it is the highest-ranking fruit source for vitamin E (yes, avocado is a fruit).
. Also, avocados are one of the best sources of monounsaturated fat, the fat known to lower artery-clogging LDL cholesterol and raise heart-healthy HDL cholesterol.

## Ingredients:

- 2 slices of whole-grain bread
- 1 avocado
- 1 pinch of sea salt
- 1 tomato

## Directions:

-1- Cut each slice of bread in half so you have 4 pieces.
-2- Put half of an avocado on one piece. Do the same for another.
-3- Add tomato slices on top.
-4- Sprinkle a tiny pinch of salt on each piece.
-5- Cover with remaining pieces of bread.

You now have two delicious, little sandwiches.

If you don't feel like having a sandwich, you can also just spread half an avocado on each slice of bread and continue the topping process from there.

## Variations:

You can add as many things as you can think of:

Blue cheese on top of the avocado
A little drop of soyonnaise
Some freshly sliced mushrooms

౮

# Goat Cheese and Berries Salad

A colorful and nutritious salad for parties!

**. Dried apricots are a great source of vitamin A.**
. Blueberries are loaded with powerful cancer-fighting antioxidants, which seem to protect vision, particularly night vision.
. If you use low-fat goat cheese, this tasty dish will contain a low level of saturated fat.
. Add vinaigrette sparingly to keep your calorie count as low as possible.

## Ingredients:

- ⅔ cup dried cranberries
- 3 tablespoons apricots, chopped and dried
- 5 tablespoons red wine vinegar (raspberry flavored is even better)
- ¼ cup of olive oil
- Salad mix (or arugula) for one regular-sized salad bowl (rinsed and crisped)
- 4 ounces of fresh goat cheese, coarsely crumbled
- 1 cup blueberries, rinsed and drained
- Salt and pepper to taste

## Directions:

-1- **Vinaigrette:** In a small microwavable bowl, combine 2 tablespoons dried cranberries, dried apricots and vinegar. Heat in microwave on high for one minute.
-2- Let stand at room temperature until cool.
-3- Put this mixture in a food processor and blend until smooth.
-4- Put back in bowl. Add oil and mix.
-5- **Salad**: In your salad bowl, combine the salad and the vinaigrette (keep 1 or 2 tablespoons of vinaigrette for decoration purposes). Mix gently.
-6- Top with crumbled cheese, blueberries and cranberries.
-7- Drizzle with remaining vinaigrette.
-8- Salt and pepper to taste.

Serves 4.

Enjoy!

∞

# Braised Cabbage

. Shiitake Mushrooms ("shii" is Japanese for "oak" and "take" means "mushroom") are delicious. They have a meaty texture and four times the flavor of white button mushrooms.
. Shiitakes provide high levels of protein (18% by mass), potassium, niacin and B vitamins, calcium, magnesium and phosphorus. Shiitake mushrooms have all essential amino acids.
. Shiitakes have natural antiviral and immunity-boosting properties, and are used nutritionally to fight viruses, lower cholesterol and regulate blood pressure.
. Mushroom protein is also superior to many other vegetable proteins due to its essential amino acid content. The white cap mushroom ranks above all other vegetables, except beans and peas in this respect. Between 70–90 percent of the vegetable protein present can be easily digested.
. Cabbage provides healthy fibers while turkey provides easily absorbable protein with a low level of saturated fat.

## Ingredients:

- 1 cabbage
- 5 shiitake mushrooms cut in 4 (can be replaced by crimini or regular white mushrooms)
- 1 clove garlic
- 250 grams ground turkey
- Soy sauce
- Margarine (non-hydrogenated)

## Directions:

-1- Shred cabbage thinly.
-2- Sauté cabbage in margarine for approx. 20 minutes on medium heat, stirring it almost NON-STOP (additional benefit: your arm will get some exercise!)
-3- Add shiitake mushrooms. Keep on low to medium heat and mix regularly while you are taking care of the next task.
-4- Grill turkey and crushed garlic in a separate skillet. Once grilled, add 2 tablespoons of soy sauce. Mix and add right away to the simmering cabbage.
-5- Mix.
-6- Reduce heat to low.
-7- Add 2 tablespoons of soy sauce. Mix.
-8- Let simmer for 20 minutes.

Enjoy!

Serves 4.

❧

# Healthy Pizza

**. A healthy way of satisfying your craving for pizza while ingesting a low amount of fat and remaining within a satisfactory Glycemic Index level.**
. Thanks to the tomato sauce, you will get plenty of cancer-fighting lycopene.
. The cheese provides necessary calcium.
. And the whole-grain bread provides iron and magnesium.

## Ingredients:

- 1 slice of whole-grain bread
- Marinara tomato sauce
- Oregano
- Olive oil
- Salt
- Shredded low-fat mozzarella or other shredded cheese (or tofu cheese)

## Directions:

**-1-** Warm up your oven to 400F.
**-2-** Put 2 tablespoons of marinara sauce on top of your slice of bread.
**-3-** Sprinkle salt (not too much) and oregano.
**-4-** Add a few drops of olive oil.
**-5-** Top with a moderate amount of shredded cheese.
**-6-** Put in the oven and take it out when cheese is bubbling on top.

Yummy!

## Variations:

You can add mushrooms and/or ham to mix things up a bit.

ॐ

# Grilled Stilton Patty

. A high-protein dish.
. If you stick to lean meat (lean beef, bison, antelope, etc.), you will keep the saturated fat content under control.

## Ingredients:

- ½ yellow onion
- 1 tablespoon canola oil
- 5 small chunks of Stilton (or any other blue cheese)
- 1 hamburger patty (beef, chicken or turkey—preferably organic)

## Directions:

-1- Peel, chop and sauté the onion in canola oil until golden-brown.
-2- In same skillet (with onions put on the side of the skillet), grill meat patty to taste (turning 3 to 4 times during cooking).
-3- When ready, turn off the heat source and place cheese chunks on top of the patty.
-4- Put a lid on the skillet to keep the heat inside.
-5- Serve when cheese is melted (2 to 3 minutes).

Serves 1.

Enjoy!

&

# Daily Fitness & Diet Log

Date [                    ]

Overall Feeling Today:   ☺ ☻ ☹     Overall Fitness:      ☺ ☻ ☹
Overall Diet:              ☺ ☻ ☹     Overall Stress Level:   ☺ ☻ ☹

## Diet...

| Breakfast | Lunch | Dinner |
|-----------|-------|--------|
| _____ | _____ | _____ |
| _____ | _____ | _____ |
| _____ | _____ | _____ |
| _____ | _____ | _____ |
| _____ | _____ | _____ |

Extra meal (if any): _____

Fluid Intake: [                ] cups. Type of fluid: _____

Trans fats?... yes / no    Refined carbs?... yes / no    Home-made food?... yes / no

## Fitness...

How many steps: [              ]

Flexibility    ☑☒: _____   🕐: _____

MetaBoost    ☑☒: _____   🕐: _____

Strength    ☑☒: _____   🕐: _____

Cardio    ☑☒: _____   🕐: _____

Other    ☑☒: _____   🕐: _____

# Day 30: BONUS DRILL
# (Days 29 & 30)

**CONGRATULATIONS ON COMPLETING "30-day BootCamp: Your
Ultimate Weight Loss Plan!"**

# It's time to CELEBRATE!

Acknowledge your success and your commitment to this program.
Relish in the fact that your clothes fit more loosely. Take pride in the
new "you," and reflect on everything you have done to stay on track with
this program.

You've done a great job!

**It is up to you now to continue eating a nutritionally-balanced diet,
with daily movement and other muscle-building activities, so that
you can maintain your goal weight, or continue releasing extra
pounds if you so choose.**

Once you have reached your ultimate goal weight, be sure to include
one or two healthy snacks (from your Snack List) to your daily diet.
Overall, listen to your body, and don't always eat when you think you
are hungry...Try a glass of water first.

## EXERCISE DRILL—Day 30—It's up to you now

Continue walking for 30 minutes every morning, on an empty stomach,
and continue getting at least 60 minutes of cumulative daily exercise.
Do at least one MetaBoost Exercise per day and you are well on your
way to healthy living and ultimate life balance.

## NUTRITIONAL TIP—Day 30—The Healthy Life

Continue eating healthy, balanced meals that include foods from all major food groups, and continue avoiding high-fat, high-sugar foods. Of course, you may enjoy your favorite foods in moderation, but be sure to eat only a small serving, rather than a large one.

One of the many goals in this BootCamp is to give you the **education and experience** you need to make healthier food choices for the rest of your life. If you revert back to your old habits, your weight will likely creep back up. To avoid that from happening, stick to the tips, move every day, and eat highly nutritious, balanced meals.

It has been a pleasure losing weight with you!

p.s. Would you like more one-on-one support with your health and fitness goals? Then, **meet your private coaches and get coached today! Just go to MyPrivateCoach.com to get started right away.**

p.s. again: I would love to hear from you. Feel free to send your thoughts and testimonials to 30daybootcamp@myprivatecoach.com. I may publish your comments in my next book (with your consent, of course) to help others on the same path.

Thank you for your participation in this program. And GOOD LUCK with all of your health and fitness goals!

Until we meet again,

*Valerie Your Private Coach*

# Daily Fitness & Diet Log

Date [                    ]

Overall Feeling Today:  ☺ ☻ ☹        Overall Fitness:        ☺ ☻ ☹
Overall Diet:           ☺ ☻ ☹        Overall Stress Level:   ☺ ☻ ☹

## Diet...

| Breakfast | Lunch | Dinner |
|-----------|-------|--------|
| _____ | _____ | _____ |
| _____ | _____ | _____ |
| _____ | _____ | _____ |
| _____ | _____ | _____ |
| _____ | _____ | _____ |

Extra meal (if any): _____

Fluid Intake: [            ] cups. Type of fluid: _____

Trans fats?... yes / no     Refined carbs?... yes / no     Home-made food?... yes / no

## Fitness...                    How many steps: [          ]

Flexibility    ☑☒: _____    🕐: _____

MetaBoost      ☑☒: _____    🕐: _____

Strength       ☑☒: _____    🕐: _____

Cardio         ☑☒: _____    🕐: _____

Other          ☑☒: _____    🕐: _____

# ଓ **Frequently Asked Questions** ଓ

**Q: What is a 30-day BootCamp?**

A: A BootCamp is an intense military training aimed at pushing people beyond their limits in order to induce change at a rapid pace. In our 30-day BootCamp, you will learn how to incorporate simple lifestyle changes and proven success habits, in order to help you lose weight FAST but in a healthy way!

It takes approximately 28 days for a new habit to develop, hence the 30-day program. After 30 days in BootCamp, you can expect to master these success habits and take them with you for the rest of your life.

**Q: How does it work?**

A: It's simple. Every day, you get a new assignment to help you accomplish your mission. These assignments include tools, exercise drills, and nutritional tips. Meanwhile, you track your progress in your daily log. Meal plans, recipes and shopping lists are also provided on a weekly basis to make this journey as simple and pain-free as possible. And, you can re-start a BootCamp as many times in the year as you wish. Is that good or is that good?

**Q: Who is my instructor?**

A: Valerie Vauthey, CEO & Founder of MyPrivatecoach.com is ready to give you the instruction, information and inspiration you need to succeed! She will help you build a healthy lifestyle that will support rapid weight loss.

Valerie has coached thousands of clients to successful weight loss, and you will see the same results, without sacrificing flavorful meals or compromising your social life.

## Q: What if the BootCamp is too hard for me?

A: No problem. Our 30-day BootCamp can be adapted to anyone's ability or commitment level. You can easily fine-tune the program to meet your needs, ability and time availability.

Of course, as in all weight loss programs, make sure you talk to your physician before embarking on a BootCamp with me.

## Q: What is a MetaBoost workout?

A: A MetaBoost is a quick, effective fitness routine, which will raise your heart rate in no time. You can easily squeeze these routines into your busy days; they are a great way to expend calories and save time. You don't have to go to a gym to do a MetaBoost workout—you can exercise in the comfort of your own home and still SEE RESULTS FAST.

## Q: Should I get my doctor's authorization?

A: As in any new diet, fitness routine, or change to your wellness program, always ask for your doctor's "okay" before starting something new. "30-day BootCamp: Your Ultimate Weight Loss Plan" provides sound, Professional information, not personalized advice. You are ultimately responsible when it comes to starting any program, so keep that in mind.

## Q: Will I have fun in BootCamp?

A: YES! Ask our BootCampers! They are raving about it. They are calling it the best-kept secret to quick weight loss without the restrictions that usually come with other "crash diet" programs. BootCamp is fun because you will discover ways to squeeze in fitness into your busy days, and you'll still enjoy your favorite foods. Everything in moderation—and the weight just keeps coming off.

## Q: Can I have pizza while in BootCamp?

YES! But I will let you find out how by reading "30-day BootCamp: Your Ultimate Weight Loss Plan." So let's get moving!

# ✂ **Resources—Summary** ✂

As you read "30-Day BootCamp: Your Ultimate Weight Loss Plan," you will have noticed that I shared several resources with you along the way.

This page summarizes all of the freebies that are mentioned throughout the book, as well as where to find the products and programs that will support your journey to a slimmer YOU.

Get your **FREE "Ultimate Daily Fitness and Diet Log"** at:
www.MyPrivateCoach.com/bootcamp_log

Get **FREE new recipes** at: www.MyPrivateCoach.com/recipes

MyPrivateCoach.com offers **Weight-Loss Coaching Programs** starting at $7/day, with a true one-on-one relationship. Make sure you visit our Weight-Loss Coaches page at: www.MyPrivateCoach.com/weightloss

You can redeem your **$50 gift certificate** at any time, for any program on www.MyPrivateCoach.com/30dayBC

**All the products I mentioned,** as well as other carefully selected top products that will support you in your slimming journey, can be found at: www.MyPrivateCoach.com/store

I would love to hear from you! Send me an e-mail with your suggestions or questions to: 30dayBootCamp@MyPrivateCoach.com

✂

# References

- Schousboe, K; Visscher, P M; Erbas; Kyvik, K O; Hopper, J L; Henriksen, J E; Heitmann, B L; Sorensen, T IA. Twin study of genetic and environmental influences on adult body size, shape, and composition. International Journal of Obesity. 28(1):39–48, January 2004.

- Mustajoki, P.; Pekkarinen, T. Very low energy diets in the treatment of obesity. Obesity Reviews. 2(1):61–72, February 2001.

- KING, NEIL ANTHONY; TREMBLAY, ANGELO; BLUNDELL, JOHN EDWARD Effects of exercise on appetite control: implications for energy balance. Medicine & Science in Sports & Exercise. 29(8):1076–1089, August 1997.

- Lange, Kai Henrik Wiborg MD; Lorentsen, Jeanne; Isaksson, Fredrik; Simonsen, Lene MD, PhD; Juul, Anders MD, PhD; Christensen, Niels Juel MD, PhD; Kjaer, Michael MD, PhD; Bulow, Jens MD, PhD. Subcutaneous Abdominal Adipose Tissue Lipolysis During Exercise Determined by Arteriovenous Measurements in Older Women. Journal of the American Geriatrics Society. 50(2):275–281, February 2002.

- NIH Consensus Development Panel. Acupuncture. *JAMA* 1998; 280:1518–1524.

- Lacey JM, Tershakovec AM, Foster GD. Acupuncture for the treatment of obesity: a review of the evidence. *International Journal of Obesity* 2003; 27:419–427.

- British Medical Association Board of Science and Education. *Acupuncture: Efficacy, Safety and Practice.* London: Harwood Academic, 2000.

- Birch S, Hesselink JK, Jonkman FA, Hekker TA, Bos A. Clinical Research on Acupuncture: Part 1. What Have Reviews of the Efficacy and Safety of Acupuncture Told Us So Far? *J Altern Complement Med.* 2004 Jun;10(3):468–80.

- Haines PS, Guilkey DK, Popkin BM: Trends in breakfast consumption of US adults between 1965 and 1991. J Am Diet Assoc 96 :464–470,1996

- Gibson SA, O'Sullivan KR: Breakfast cereal consumption patterns and nutrient intakes of British schoolchildren. J R Soc Health 115 :336–370,1995 .

- Summerbell CD, Moody RC, Shanks J, Stock MJ, Geissler C: Relationship between feeding pattern and body mass index in 220 free-living people in four age groups. Eur J Clin Nutr50 :513–519,1996.

- Ortega RM, Requejo AM, Lopez-Sobaler AM, Quintas ME, Andres P, Redondo MR, Navia B, Lopez-Bonilla MD, Rivas T: Differences in the breakfast habits of overweight/obese and normal weight schoolchildren. Int J Vitam Nutr Res68 :125–132,1998.

- Bellisle F, Rolland-Cachera MF, Deheeger M, Guilloud-Bataille M: Obesity and food intake in children: evidence for a role of metabolic and/or behavioral daily rhythms. Appetite 11 :111–118,1988.

- Ortega RM, Redondo MR, Lopez-Sobaler AM, Quintas ME, Zamora MJ, Andres P, Encinas-Sotillos A: Associations between obesity, breakfast-time food habits and intake of energy and nutrients in a group of elderly Madrid residents. J Am Coll Nutr15 :65–72,1996.

- Wolfe WS, Campbell CC, Frongillo EA, Haas JD, Melnick TA: Overweight schoolchildren in New York state: prevalence and characteristics. Am J Public Health84 :807–813,1994

- Keim NL, Van Loan MD, Horn WF, Barbieri TF, Mayclin PL: Weight loss is greater with consumption of large morning meals and fat-free mass is preserved with large evening meals in women on a controlled weight reduction regimen. J Nutr 127 :75–82,1997

- Nicklas, TA, Myers, L, Reger, C, Beech, B, Berenson, GS (1998) Impact of breakfast consumption on nutritional adequacy of the diets of young adults in Bogalusa, Louisiana: ethnic and gender contrasts J Am Diet Assoc 98,1432–1438

- Zabik, ME (1987) Impact of ready-to-eat cereal consumption on nutrient intake Cereal Foods World 32,234–9

- Schlundt DG, Hill JO, Sbrocco T, Pope-Cordle J, Sharp T: The role of breakfast in the treatment of obesity: a randomized clinical trial. Am J Clin Nutr 55 :645–651,1992

- Morgan, KJ, Zabik, ME, Stampley, GL (1986) The role of breakfast in the diet adequacy of the US population J Am Coll Nutr 5,551–563

- Martin A, Normand S, Sothier M, Peyrat J, Louche-Pelissier C, Laville M: Is advice for breakfast consumption justified? Results from a short-term dietary and metabolic experiment in young healthy men. Br J Nutr 84 :337–344,2000

- Cho S, Dietrich M, Brown CJ, Clark CA, Block G.The effect of breakfast type on total daily energy intake and body mass index: results from the Third National Health and Nutrition Examination Survey (NHANES III). J Am Coll Nutr. 2003 Aug;22(4):296–302.

- Ma Y, Bertone ER, Stanek EJ 3rd, Reed GW, Hebert JR, Cohen NL, Merriam PA, Ockene IS. Association between eating patterns and obesity in a free-living US adult population. Am J Epidemiol. 2003 Jul 1;158(1):85–92.

- Berkey CS, Rockett HR, Gillman MW, Field AE, Colditz GA. Longitudinal study of skipping breakfast and weight change in adolescents. Int J Obes Relat Metab Disord. 2003 Oct;27(10):1258–66.

- Fugh-Berman, Adriane MD, Reviewer Health Food Junkies: Orthorexia Nervosa: Overcoming the Obsession With Healthful Eating. JAMA. msJAMA. 285(17):2255–2256, May 2, 2001.

- Bidoli, E. et al (1992), Food consumption and cancer of the colon and rectum in North-Eastern Italy, International Jnl of Cancer v.50 p.223–229.

- Ling, W. Shifting from a Conventional Diet to an Uncooked Vegan Diet Reversibly Alters Fecal Hydrolytic Activities in Humans. Journal of Nutrition, 122: 924–930,1992.

- Kjeldsen-Kragh, J. Controlled trial of fasting and one-year vegetarian diet in rheumatoid arthritis. Lancet, 1991; 338:899–902.

- Rao, A V. & Janezic, S A. (1992), The role of dietary phyosterols in colon carcinogenesis, Nutrition & Cancer v.18 (1) p.43–52.

- Knoops, Kim T. B. MSc; de Groot, Lisette C. P. G. M. PhD; Kromhout, Daan PhD; Perrin, Anne-Elisabeth MD, MSc; Moreiras-Varela, Olga PhD; Menotti, Alessandro MD, PhD; van Staveren, Wija A. PhD Mediterranean Diet, Lifestyle Factors, and 10-Year Mortality in Elderly European Men and Women: The HALE Project. JAMA. 292(12):1433–1439, September 22/29, 2004.

- Girois, Susan B. MD; Kumanyika, Shiriki K. PhD, MPH; Morabia, Alfredo MD, PhD, MPH; Mauger, Elizabeth PhD A Comparison of Knowledge and Attitudes About Diet and Health Among 35- to 75-Year-Old Adults in the United States and Geneva, Switzerland. American Journal of Public Health. Risky Concepts: Methods in Cancer Research. 91(3):418–424, March 2001.

- Pearce, Neil professor; Foliaki, Sunia research fellow; Sporle, Andrew research fellow; Cunningham, Chris professor. Genetics, race, ethnicity, and health. BMJ. 328(7447):1070–1072, May 1, 2004.

- Diamond, Jared The double puzzle of diabetes. Nature. 423(6940):599–602, June 5, 2003.

- Rutten, A ; Ziemainz, H; Schena, F; Stahl, T; Stiggelbout, M; Auweele, Y Vanden; Vuillemin, A; Welshman, J. Using different physical activity measurements in eight European countries. Results of the European Physical Activity Surveillance System (EUPASS) time series survey. Public Health Nutrition. 6(4):371–376, June 2003.

- Greenwood CE, McGee CD, Dyer JR. Influence of dietary fat on brain membrane phospholipid fatty acid composition and neuronal function in mature rats. Nutrition 1989;5:278–81.

- Farquarson J, Cockburn F, Patrick WA, Jamieson EC, Logan RW. Infant cerebral cortex phospholipid fatty-acid composition and diet. Lancet 1992; 340:810–3.

- Stoll AL, Severus WE, Freeman MP, Rueter S, Zboyan HA, Diamond E, et al. Omega 3 fatty acids in bipolar disorder: a preliminary double-blind, placebo-controlled trial. Arch Gen Psychiatry 1999;56(5):407–12.

- Spring BJ, Lieberman HR, Swope G, Garfield GS. Effects of carbohydrates on mood and behavior. Nutr Rev 1986;44:51–60.

- Craig A. Acute effects of meals on perceptual and cognitive efficiency. Nutr Rev 1986;44(Suppl):163–71.

- Young, Simon N. Clinical nutrition: 3. The fuzzy boundary between nutrition and psychopharmacology. CMAJ Canadian Medical Association Journal. 166(2):205–209, January 22, 2002.

- Gold PE. Role of glucose in regulating the brain and cognition. Am J Clin Nutr 1995;61:S987–95.

- Wolraich ML, Lindgren SD, Stumbo PJ, Stegink LD, Appelbaum MI, Kiritsy MC. Effects of diets high in sucrose or aspartame on the behavior and cognitive performance of children. N Engl J Med 1994;330:301–7.

- Wolraich ML, Wilson DB, White JW. The effect of sugar on behavior or cognition in children: a meta-analysis. JAMA 1995;274:1617–21.

- Polivy, Janet 1,2; Herman, C Peter 1 If at First You Don't Succeed: False Hopes of Self-Change. American Psychologist. 57(9):677–689, September 2002.

- Stice, Eric 1,2; Mazotti, Lindsay 1; Krebs, Melora 1; Martin, Sarah 1 Predictors of Adolescent Dieting Behaviors: A Longitudinal Study. Psychology of Addictive Behaviors. 12(3):195–205, September 1998.

- Luckman, Simon M Is There Such a Thing as a Healthy Appetite?. Journal of Neuroendocrinology. 13(9):739–740, September 2001.

- Brachfeld, Jonas MD The Obesity Epidemic. Archives of Internal Medicine. 164(18):2066, October 11, 2004.

- WALKER, A. R.P. With increasing ageing in Western populations, what are the prospects for lowering the incidence of coronary heart disease? Qjm. 94(2):107–112, February 2001.

- Swinburn, Boyd; Egger, Garry. The runaway weight gain train: too many accelerators, not enough brakes. BMJ. 329(7468):736–739, September 25, 2004.

- Coffey, C S; Steiner, D; Baker, B A; Allison, D B. A randomized double-blind placebo-controlled clinical trial of a product containing ephedrine, caffeine, and other ingredients from herbal sources for treatment of overweight and obesity in the absence of lifestyle treatment. International Journal of Obesity. 28(11):1411–1419, November 2004.

- Hamilton, M.; Greenway, F. Evaluating commercial weight loss programmes: an evolution in outcomes research. Obesity Reviews. 5(4):217–232, November 2004.

- Bravata, Dena M. MD, MS; Sanders, Lisa MD; Huang, Jane MD; Krumholz, Harlan M. MD, SM; Olkin, Ingram PhD; Gardner, Christopher D. PhD; Bravata, Dawn M. MD Efficacy and Safety of Low-Carbohydrate Diets: A Systematic Review. JAMA. 289(14):1837–1850, April 9, 2003.

- Irwin, Melinda L.; Yasui, Yutaka; Ulrich, Cornelia M.; Bowen, Deborah; Rudolph, Rebecca E.; Schwartz, Robert S.; Yukawa, Michi; Aiello, Erin; Potter, John D.; McTiernan, Anne Effect of Exercise on Total and Intraabdominal Body Fat in Postmenopausal Women: A Randomized, Controlled Trial. Obstetrical & Gynecological Survey. 58(7):469–470, July 2003.

- Lara-Castro, Cristina; Garvey, W Timothy Diet, Insulin Resistance, and Obesity: Zoning in on Data for Atkins Dieters Living in South Beach. Journal of Clinical Endocrinology & Metabolism. 89(9):4197–4205, September 2004.

- Bray GA, Popkin BM. Dietary fat intake does affect obesity!Am J Clin Nutr 1998;68:1157–73.

- Astrup A, Grunwald GK, Melanson EL, *et al.* The role of low-fat diets in body weight control: a meta-analysis of ad libitum dietary intervention studies. *Int J Obes Relat Metab Disord* 2000;24:1545–52.

- Kopelman, P G 1; Grace, C 2 New thoughts on managing obesity. Gut. 53(7):1044–1053, July 2004.

- Kirk TR. Role of dietary carbohydrate and frequent eating in body-weight control.

Proc Nutr Soc. 2000 Aug;59(3):349–58

- Astrup A, Ryan L, Grunwald GK, Storgaard M, Saris W, Melanson E, Hill JO. The role of dietary fat in body fatness: evidence from a preliminary meta-analysis of ad libitum low-fat dietary intervention studies. Br J Nutr. 2000 Mar;83 Suppl 1:S25–32.

- Jequier E. Pathways to obesity. Int J Obes Relat Metab Disord. 2002 Sep;26 Suppl 2:S12–7.

- GD Foster, HR Wyatt, JO Hill et al., A randomized trial of a low-carbohydrate diet for obesity. N Engl J Med 348 (2003), pp. 2082–2090.

- L Stern, N Iqbal, P Seshadri et al., The effects of low-carbohydrate versus conventional weight loss diets in severely obese adults: one-year follow-up of a randomized trial. Ann Intern Med 140 (2004), pp. 778–785.

- Whitney, E. N., and S. R. Rolfes. Understanding Nutrition. Belmont, CA: West/Wadsworth, 1999, pp. 215–238, 443–447.

- Symons JD, Jacobs I. High-intensity exercise performance is not impaired by low intramuscular glycogen. Med Sci Sports Exerc. 1989 Oct;21(5):550–7.

- Eva Blomstrand and Bengt Saltin. Effect of muscle glycogen on glucose, lactate and amino acid metabolism during exercise and recovery in human subjects. J Appl Physiol 514.1: 293–302, 1999.

- Pietro Galassetti, Stephnie Mann, Donna Tate, Ray A. Neill, David H. Wasserman, and Stephen N. Davis. Effect of morning exercise on counterregulatory responses to subsequent, afternoon exercise. J Appl Physiol 91: 91–99, 2001.

- Echwald, S. M. Genetics of human obesity: lessons from mouse models and candidate genes. *Journal of Internal Medicine. 245(6):653–666, June 1999.*

- Spiegelman BM, Flier JS 2001 Obesity and the regulation of energy balance. Cell 104: 531–543.

- Rosenbaum, Michael; Leibel, Rudolph L.; Hirsch, Jules Medical Progress: Obesity. *New England Journal of Medicine. 337(6):396–407, August 7, 1997.*

- Tremblay A, Buemann B. Exercise-training, macronutrient balance and body weight control. Int J Obes Relat Metab Disord 1995;19:79–86.

- Weintraub M. Long-term weight control study: conclusions. Clin Pharmacol Ther 1992;51:642–6.

- Brownell KD, Fairburn CG, eds. Eating disorders and obesity: a comprehensive handbook. New York: Guilford Press, 1995.

- Petibois, Cyril; Cassaigne, Andre; Gin, Henri; Deleris, Gerard Lipid Profile Disorders Induced by Long-Term Cessation of Physical Activity in Previously Highly Endurance-Trained Subjects. Journal of Clinical Endocrinology & Metabolism. 89(7):3377–3384, July 2004.

- Berggren, Jason R; Hulver, Matthew W; Dohm, G Lynis; Houmard, Joseph A. Weight Loss and Exercise: Implications for Muscle Lipid Metabolism and Insulin Action. Medicine & Science in Sports & Exercise. 36(7):1191–1195, July 2004.

- Goodpaster, Bret H.; Katsiaras, Andreas; Kelley, David E. Enhanced Fat Oxidation Through Physical Activity Is Associated With Improvements in Insulin Sensitivity in Obesity. Diabetes. 52(9):2191–2197, September 2003.

- Abdel-Hamid, T. Modeling the dynamics of human energy regulation and its implications for obesity treatment. System Dynamics Rev. 18: 431–471, 2002.

- Abdul-Hamid, Tarek K. Exercise and Diet in Obesity Treatment: An Integrative System Dynamics Perspective. Medicine & Science in Sports & Exercise. 35(3):400–413, March 2003.

- Goodpaster, Bret H.; Katsiaras, Andreas; Kelley, David E. Enhanced Fat Oxidation Through Physical Activity Is Associated With Improvements in Insulin Sensitivity in Obesity. Diabetes. 52(9):2191–2197, September 2003.

- Thornton, Kathleen; Potteiger, Jeffery A. Effects of resistance exercise bouts of different intensities but equal work on EPOC. Medicine & Science in Sports & Exercise. 34(4):715–722, April 2002.

- Bell, Christopher; Day, Danielle S.; Jones, Pamela P.; Christou, Demetra D.; Petitt, Darby S.; Osterberg, Kris; Melby, Christopher L.; Seals, Douglas R. High Energy Flux Mediates the Tonically Augmented [beta]-Adrenergic Support of Resting Metabolic Rate in Habitually Exercising Older Adults. Journal of Clinical Endocrinology & Metabolism. 89(7):3573–3578, July 2004.

- Cullum, Mark G. 1; Pittsley, Jesse 2; Yates, James W. FACSM 2 The Variability of Resting Metabolic Rate Measurements. Medicine & Science in Sports & Exercise. 36(5) Supplement:S247, May 2004.

- Mikat, Richard P. Correlation of Intake Frequency, Resting Metabolic Rate and Body Mass Index in Women. Medicine & Science in Sports & Exercise. 36(5) Supplement:S97, May 2004.

- Buchheit, Martin; Simon, Chantal; Viola, Antoine Uranio; Doutreleau, Stephanie; Piquard, Francois; Brandenberger, Gabrielle. Heart Rate Variability in Sportive Elderly: Relationship with Daily Physical Activity. Medicine & Science in Sports & Exercise. 36(4):601–605, April 2004.

- Bell, Christopher; Jones, Pamela P.; Seals, Douglas R. Oxidative Stress Does Not Modulate Metabolic Rate or Skeletal Muscle Sympathetic Activity with Primary Aging in Adult Humans. Journal of Clinical Endocrinology & Metabolism. 88(10):4950–4954, October 2003.

- Ormsbee, M J. 1; Martin-Pressman, R 1; Everett, M 1; Zwicky, L 1; Cogan, G 1; Arciero, P J. Facsm 1 effects of aerobic and resistance training on body composition, RMR, blood lipids, and muscular strength training in middle-aged women and men. Medicine & Science in Sports & Exercise. 35(5) Supplement 1:S33, May 2003.

- Abdul-Hamid, Tarek K. Exercise and Diet in Obesity Treatment: An Integrative System Dynamics Perspective. Medicine & Science in Sports & Exercise. 35(3):400–413, March 2003.

- Petibois, Cyril; Cassaigne, Andre; Gin, Henri; Deleris, Gerard Lipid Profile Disorders Induced by Long-Term Cessation of Physical Activity in Previously Highly Endurance-Trained Subjects. Journal of Clinical Endocrinology & Metabolism. 89(7):3377–3384, July 2004.

- Berggren, Jason; Hluver, Matthew; Dohm, G; Lynis; Houmard, Joseph A.Weight Loss and Exercise: Implications for Muscle Lipid Metabolism and Insulin Action. Medicine & Science in Sports & Exercise. 36(7):1191–1195, July 2004.

- Whitney, E. N., and S. R. Rolfes. Understanding Nutrition. Belmont, CA: West/Wadsworth, 1999, pp. 215–238, 443–447.

- Goodpaster, Bret H.; Katsiaras, Andreas; Kelley, David E. Enhanced Fat Oxidation Through Physical Activity Is Associated With Improvements in Insulin Sensitivity in Obesity. Diabetes. 52(9):2191–2197, September 2003.

978-0-595-38006-0
0-595-38006-9

Made in the USA